D0992036

AGE AND
THE PHARMACOLOGY
OF PSYCHOACTIVE DRUGS

AGE AND
THE PHARMACOLOGY
OF PSYCHOACTIVE DRUGS

Editors-in-Chief

ALLEN RASKIN, Ph. D.
Chief, Anxiety Disorders Section
Pharmacologic and Somatic Treatments Branch
National Institute of Mental Health
Rockville, Maryland

DONALD S. ROBINSON, M.D.
Chairman, Department of Pharmacology
Marshall University School of Medicine
Huntington, West Virginia

JEROME LEVINE, M.D.
Chief, Pharmacologic and Somatic Treatments Branch
National Institute of Mental Health
Rockville, Maryland

ELSEVIER
New York • Oxford

Elsevier North Holland, Inc.
52 Vanderbilt Avenue, New York, New York 10017

Sole distributors outside USA and Canada:
Elsevier Science Publishers B.V.
P.O. Box 211, 1000 AE Amsterdam, The Netherlands

Library of Congress Cataloging in Publication Data

Main entry under title:

Age and the pharmacology of psychoactive drugs.

  Includes bibliographies and index.
  1. Psychopharmacology. 2. Geriatric pharmacology. 3. Pediatric
pharmacology. I. Raskin, Allen, 1926– II. Robinson, Donald
S. III. Levine, Jerome, 1934– [DNLM: 1. Drug therapy—In infancy
and childhood. 2. Drug therapy—In old age. 3. Psychotropic drugs—
Pharmacodynamics. QV 77 A266]
RM315.A44   615′.78   81-9749
ISBN 0-444-00586-2   AACR2

Desk Editor John Haber
Design Edmée Froment
Design Editors Glen Burris and Aimee Kudlak
Production Manager Joanne Jay
Compositor Ampersand, Inc.
Printer Haddon Craftsmen

Manufactured in the United States of America

CONTENTS

PREFACE

Until recent years little was known or appreciated about age-related changes in the pharmacokinetics and pharmacodynamics of drugs, especially the psychoactive agents. The importance of this problem in clinical therapeutics is now recognized widely, but considerable work still needs to be done.

This book aims to bridge the gap between basic and applied psychopharmacology with special reference to both ends of the age spectrum, i.e., children and the elderly. The idea for this book grew out of informal discussions among ourselves and others indicating there were important similarities and differences in the pharmacodynamics and pharmacokinetics of psychoactive drugs in both the very young and the very old; these differences and similarities could have important implications for medication management in these age groups. A developmental approach to the pharmacology of psychoactive drugs has also not had a clear emphasis or focus in prior publications. However, before launching into a book on this topic it was decided to bring experts together from the fields of pediatric, geriatric, and adult psychopharmacology, as well as experts in basic psychopharmacology, to exchange information and ideas in a workshop setting. That meeting took place in Washington, D.C., in April 1979 and was quite successful in providing a forum for an exchange of information and in stimulating interest among the participants in the general theme of age-related changes in the pharmacology of psychoactive drugs. Following the meeting a majority of the speakers were willing to expand the papers they had presented into chapters for this book. We also solicited a number of additional chapters to cover topics whose importance became apparent during or after the discussions.

The book is divided into two major sections: The first, Basic Pharmacodynamic and Pharmacokinetic Issues, provides an overview of critical issues regarding the influence of age on neural transmission (J.T. Coyle and M.V. Johnston), on the blood–brain barrier (S.I. Rapoport), on monoamine oxidase (MAO) levels in body tissues (T.P. Bridge and associates), on biogenic amine synthesis (R.A. Levine and associates), on pharmacokinetic factors such as drug binding and distribution (G.R. Wilkinson), and on the hyperkinetic syndrome (G. Breese and others).

Chapter 7, by T.F. Blaschke, provides a transition between the basic and more applied sections of the book. This chapter builds on the changes in basic pharmacodynamics and pharmacokinetics associated with aging and shows how these factors modify and often increase liability for drug toxicity in elderly patients. Four chapters are devoted to the antidepressant drugs; this is because the amount of information available on the pharmacokinetics of antidepressants and on antidepressant drug use in both children and the elderly is much larger than for other psychoactive drugs. Three chapters are devoted to the tricyclic antidepressants (TCAs): J.L. Rapoport and W.Z. Potter describe their use in children, R.O. Friedel focuses on TCA use in the elderly, and J.J. Schildkraut discusses the former two chapters and also discusses special issues such as differences in TCA pharmacology following chronic versus acute drug administration. The monoamine oxidase inhibitors (MAOIs) are receiving increasing attention for treating depression in the elderly because of the interesting finding that MAO levels increase with age. There is also some recent evidence that MAOIs may be more efficacious in older than in younger patients. D.S. Robinson is a pioneer in this field, and his chapter focuses on MAOI use in the elderly.

The remaining chapters in the second section of the book discuss changes in pharmacokinetics associated with age in relation to other classes of psychoactive drugs, such as lithium (R.F. Prien), the psychostimulants (C. Salzman), and the neuroleptics (T.B. Cooper and D.S. Robinson). R.F. Prien's chapter describes lithium usage in children and the elderly; the chapters on the psychostimulants and neuroleptics focus exclusively on the elderly.

The final section of the book, Overview and Future Directions, is a chapter by Folke Sjöqvist. We were fortunate that Dr. Sjöqvist was spending a sabbatical year at the National Institutes of Health in Washington, D.C., and so was available to attend the April 1979 workshop. Dr. Sjöqvist was the final speaker at that workshop and summed up the state of the art as reflected by the workshop presentations and discussions. His chapter is essentially an elaboration of his remarks at the workshop, but it also includes references to and descriptions of his own work that illustrate the direction in which he believes the field should be moving.

To the extent that we were successful in bridging the gap between basic and applied psychopharmacology, this book should have added appeal to psychopharmacology practitioners and researchers. The developmental approach of this book is unique and should be of special interest to those involved in pediatric and geriatric psychopharmacology. It was also our fervent wish that this book would stimulate other investigators to examine age-related or developmental changes in their own work and to relate their findings to practical issues of psychoactive drug management in young and old patients.

We would be remiss if we did not take this opportunity to thank all those who contributed to this volume. It was our impression that many contributors were willing to take the time from their busy schedules to prepare these chapters because of the challenge posed of conceptualizing their own work and the work of others into a developmental framework. We also want to thank the numerous individuals at the National Institute of Mental Health (NIMH) who provided support and encouragement for the April 1979 workshop and for this book. We would like to mention in this regard Louis A. Wienckowski, Director of the Division of Extramural Research Programs, James E. Moynihan, the Associate Director of that Division, and Nancy K. Cahill, Administrative Officer. Special thanks are also in order to Diane Cheslosky, who prepared correspondence, proofed and retyped manuscripts, and performed many other functions essential to the preparation of this book.

ALLEN RASKIN
DONALD S. ROBINSON
JEROME LEVINE

CONTRIBUTORS

TERRANCE F. BLASCHKE, M.D.
Chief, Division of Clinical Pharmacology, Stanford University, Palo Alto, California

GEORGE BREESE, Ph.D.
Professor of Pharmacology and Psychiatry, Biological Sciences Research Center, University of North Carolina School of Medicine, Chapel Hill, North Carolina

T. PETER BRIDGE, M.D.
Research Psychiatrist, Laboratory of Clinical Psychopharmacology, Division of Special Mental Health Research, Intramural Research Program, National Institute of Mental Health, Saint Elizabeth's Hospital, Washington, D.C.

THOMAS B. COOPER
Principal Research Scientist, Analytical Psychopharmacology Laboratory, Rockland Research Institute, Orangeburg, New York

JOSEPH T. COYLE, M.D.
Associate Professor of Pharmacology and Psychiatry, Departments of Pharmacology and Experimental Therapeutics and Psychiatry and the Behavioral Sciences, Johns Hopkins University School of Medicine, Baltimore, Maryland

ROBERT O. FRIEDEL, M.D.
Professor and Chairman, Department of Psychiatry, Medical College of Virginia, Virginia Commonwealth University, Richmond, Virginia

THOMAS GUALTIERI, M.D.
Assistant Professor of Psychiatry, Biological Sciences Research Center, University of North Carolina School of Medicine, Chapel Hill, North Carolina

MICHAEL V. JOHNSTON, M.D.
Departments of Pharmacology and Experimental Therapeutics and Psychiatry and the Behavioral Sciences, Johns Hopkins University School of Medicine, Baltimore, Maryland

DONALD M. KUHN, Ph.D.
Senior Staff Fellow, Section on Biochemical Pharmacology, National Heart, Lung, and Blood Institute, National Institutes of Health, Bethesda, Maryland

JEROME LEVINE, M.D.
Chief, Pharmacologic and Somatic Treatments Branch, National Institute of Mental Health, Rockville, Maryland

ROBERT A. LEVINE
Section on Biochemical Pharmacology, National Heart, Lung, and Blood Institute, National Institutes of Health, Bethesda, Maryland

WALTER LOVENBERG, Ph.D.
Head of Section on Biochemical Pharmacology, National Heart, Lung, and Blood Institute, National Institutes of Health, Bethesda, Maryland

RICHARD MAILMAN, Ph.D.
Research Associate Professor, Departments of Psychiatry and Pharmacology, Biological Sciences Research Center, University of North Carolina School of Medicine, Chapel Hill, North Carolina

ROBERT MUELLER, M.D.
Departments of Anesthesiology and Pharmacology, Biological Sciences Research Center, University of North Carolina School of Medicine, Chapel Hill, North Carolina

BRUCE H. PHELPS, Ph.D.
Staff Fellow, Laboratory of Clinical Psychopharmacology, Division of Special Mental Health Research, Intramural Research Program, National Institute of Mental Health, Saint Elizabeth's Hospital, Washington, D.C.

STEVEN POTKIN, M.D.
Research Psychiatrist, Laboratory of Clinical Psychopharmacology, Division of Special Mental Health Research, Intramural Research Program, National Institute of Mental Health, Saint Elizabeth's Hospital, Washington, D.C.

WILLIAM Z. POTTER, M.D., Ph.D.
Assistant to the Branch Chief, Clinical Psychobiology Branch, National Institute of Mental Health and Coordinator for Clinical Pharmacology, National Institute of General Medical Sciences, Bethesda, Maryland

ROBERT F. PRIEN, Ph.D.
Chief, Affective Disorders Section, Pharmacologic and Somatic Treatments Branch, National Institute of Mental Health, Rockville, Maryland

JUDITH L. RAPOPORT, M.D.
Chief, Unit on Childhood Mental Illness, National Institue of Mental Health, Bethesda, Maryland

STANLEY I. RAPOPORT, M.D.
Chief, Laboratory of Neurosciences, National Institute on Aging, Gerontology Research Center, Baltimore City Hospitals, Baltimore, Maryland

ALLEN RASKIN, Ph.D.
Chief, Anxiety Disorders Section, Pharmacologic and Somatic Treatments Branch, National Institute of Mental Health, Rockville, Maryland

DONALD S. ROBINSON, M.D.
Chairman, Department of Pharmacology, Marshall University School of Medicine, Huntington, West Virginia

CARL SALZMAN, M.D.
Associate Professor of Psychiatry, Harvard Medical School, Massachusetts Mental Health Center, Boston, Massachusetts

JOSEPH J. SCHILDKRAUT, M.D.
Professor of Psychiatry, Harvard Medical School, Massachusetts Mental Health Center, Boston, Massachusetts

FOLKE SJÖQVIST, M.D.
Professor, Department of Clincial Pharmacology at the Karolinska Institute, Huddinge Hospital, S-14186 Huddinge, Sweden

RICHARD VOGEL, Ph.D.
Research Fellow, Biological Sciences Research Center, University of North Carolina School of Medicine, Chapel Hill, North Carolina

GRANT R. WILKINSON, Ph.D.
Department of Pharmacology, Vanderbilt University School of Medicine, Nashville, Tennessee

ADRIAN C. WILLIAMS, M.D.
Visiting Associate, Section on Biochemical Pharmacology, National Heart, Lung, and Blood Institute, National Institutes of Health, Bethesda, Maryland

JANET WILSON, B.S.
Research Assistant, Biological Sciences Research Center, University of North Carolina School of Medicine, Chapel Hill, North Carolina

C. DAVID WISE, Ph.D.
Staff Fellow, Laboratory of Clinical Psychopharmacology, Division of Special Mental Health Research, Intramural Research Program, National Institute of Mental Health, Saint Elizabeth's Hospital, Washington, D.C.

RICHARD JED WYATT, M.D.
Director, Laboratory of Clinical Psychopharmacology, Division of Special Mental Health Research, Intramural Research Program, National Institute of Mental Health, Saint Elizabeth's Hospital, Washington, D.C.

WILLIAM YOUNGBLOOD, Ph.D.
Research Associate Professor of Biochemistry, Biological Sciences Research Center, University of North Carolina School of Medicine, Chapel Hill, North Carolina

I

BASIC PHARMACODYNAMIC AND PHARMACOKINETIC ISSUES

1

EFFECTS OF AGING ON THE DISPOSITION OF BENZODIAZEPINES IN HUMAN BEINGS:
BINDING AND DISTRIBUTION CONSIDERATIONS

G. R. Wilkinson

The potential for altered drug responsiveness in the elderly is well recognized, although the almost twofold greater incidence of adverse reactions in this population (17) is an indication of the practical difficulties involved in compensating for such changes. Differences in the way the drug is handled by the body and alterations in drug–receptor interactions at the effector site may all be responsible for such a phenomenon. Unfortunately, knowledge in either area is extremely meager, although more is known concerning age-related differences in the pharmacokinetic factors than of the pharmacodynamic ones.

Generally, comparative pharmacokinetic studies in the young and elderly have depended on concentration/time profiles of the total amount of drug in the circulation. However, it is now appreciated that the various processes of drug disposition often depend on the circulating concentration of unbound or "free" drug, i.e., that not associated with various macromolecules such as albumin, α_1 acid glycoprotein, and lipoproteins. Moreover, it is generally assumed that only unbound drug can cross membranes to reach the sites of drug action. Therefore, this chapter reviews briefly the effects of aging on drug binding and the consequences of this on the disposition of several benzodiazepines.

PHARMACOKINETIC CONSIDERATIONS OF PLASMA AND TISSUE BINDING

Because membranes are only permeable to unbound drug moieties, it has frequently been assumed that drug binding in the blood limits the rate of

From the Department of Pharmacology, Vanderbilt University School of Medicine, Nashville, Tennessee. Supported by United States Public Health Service grants GM 15431 and AG 01395.

drug elimination by organs such as the liver and kidney. While a proportionality between binding and clearance may exist, as exemplified by glomerular filtration, consideration of organ transit times and dissociation rate constants for drug-protein complexes indicates that this may not always occur (10). In fact, there are examples in which renal or hepatic extraction is greater than the free fraction present in the delivered blood, implying that the drug must be "stripped" from its binding sites during passage through the organ.

To account for these different findings, a modification of the venous equilibration or well-stirred model of organ extraction (31) was suggested for linear conditions, i.e., neither binding nor metabolism is saturable (34, 41), as indicated in equations (1) and (2).

$$\text{extraction} = E = \frac{f_B Cl'_{int}}{Q + f_B Cl'_{int}} \tag{1}$$

$$\text{clearance} = QE = Q \left[\frac{f_B Cl'_{int}}{Q + f_B Cl'_{int}} \right] \tag{2}$$

where Cl'_{int} is the free intrinsic clearance of drug from the organ's intracellular water, Q is total organ blood flow, and f_B is the fraction of drug unbound in the blood ($f_B = f_P / (B/P)$, where f_P is the free fraction in the plasma and B/P is the drug's blood/plasma concentration ratio). According to these relationships, when extraction is small compared to Cl'_{int}/Q then an approximate proportionality exists across the whole binding range (Figure 1). Accordingly, extraction/clearance increases almost linearly with f_B, as exemplified by the findings with warfarin (24). However, as the organ's intrinsic ability to eliminate drug increases a curvilinear relationship develops and the extraction ratio may become greater than the free fraction (Figure 1). In fact, in this situation binding in the blood functions as a delivery system augmenting drug elimination. The clearance of propranolol appears to fit this type of behavior (34).

It would be expected a priori that binding in the blood would affect drug distribution out of the vascular space independently. This may be appreciated by the quantitative approach of Gillette (10) to the volume of distribution (Vd) as shown in equation (3).

$$\text{Vd} = V_B + V_T(f_B / f_T) \tag{3}$$

where V_B is the blood volume, V_T is the volume of the other tissues of the body, and f_T and f_B are fractions of drug present in the unbound form in tissue and blood, respectively. Thus, with an increase in free fraction, the volume of distribution increases from the limiting value of the blood volume to an infinitely large volume determined by the ratio of the free fraction in blood and tissue (Figure 2) (41). It also follows that if tissue

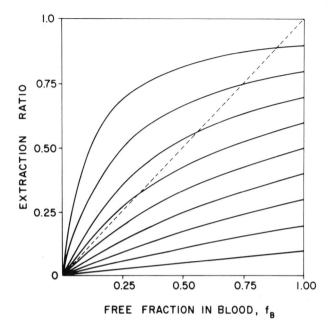

FIGURE 1. Effect of binding in the blood on organ extraction ratio. Dashed line indicates when $E = f_B$; below this line extraction is limited to the unbound moiety, whereas above the line bound drug delivered to the organ is extracted. Each curve represents different values of Cl'_{int}/Q corresponding to 10% step-wise changes in extraction when $f_B = 1$. (From Ref. [41].)

binding is changed, Vd will be altered, and a perturbation in blood binding may not necessarily lead to a change in the volume distribution if tissue binding is also affected so that the ratio f_B/f_T remains constant (8).

Both systemic clearance (Cl_S) and volume of distribution are important pharmacokinetic parameters determined by physiologic factors (equations [2] and [3]). Their interaction leads to another important but empirical value, the elimination half-life (equation 4).

$$t_{1/2} = 0.693 Vd/Cl_S \qquad (4)$$

If only a single organ is involved in the elimination process, i.e., liver or kidneys, substitution of equations (2) and (3) and simplification (41) leads to the following relationship:

$$t_{1/2} = 0.693 \left[\frac{Vd}{Q} + \frac{Vd}{f_B Cl'_{int}} \right] \qquad (5)$$

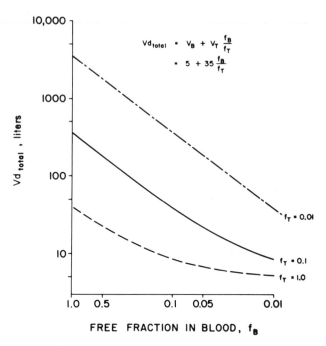

$$Vd_{total} = V_B + V_T \frac{f_B}{f_T}$$

$$= 5 + 35 \frac{f_B}{f_T}$$

FREE FRACTION IN BLOOD, f_B

FIGURE 2. Effect of altering the fraction of binding in the blood on the volume of distribution of total drug. The three curves represent different degrees of tissue binding $(1 - f_T)$. (From Ref. [41].)

More complex equations may be developed for situations in which more than one organ is responsible for drug elimination, e.g., both liver and kidneys. Based on equation (5) the effects of binding in the blood on the rate of elimination may be visualized as the sum of two tendencies; with a decrease in free fraction in blood the left-hand term will lead to a decrease in half-life, whereas the right-hand term will tend to increase half-life. Thus as f_B decreases from unity, the half-life decreases to a minimum, then increases to become infinitely long when all the drug is bound in the blood. The precise change is dependent on the free intrinsic clearance and the degree of tissue binding (41). In general, for drugs with a small clearance and volume of distribution the shortening in half-life is barely detectable, and binding changes produce a proportional prolongation of the half-life; whereas for a drug with the opposite characteristics, such as propranolol, an increase in binding leads to a shortened half-life (7).

It is also important to consider the effect of binding in the blood on the concentration/time relationship following drug administration. This relationship is obviously controlled by the previously considered pharmacokinetic parameters. A convenient parameter that integrates them all is the total area under the blood concentration/time curve (the area under the curve [AUC]). The AUC may be estimated following acute drug administration or chronic dosing, since in the latter case the AUC is related proportionally to the average steady-state blood level by the dosage interval. Hence the effects of binding differences following acute and steady-state dosing can both be considered. Even if the drug is metabolized by the liver only following complete absorption of the administered dose (D) the situation is fairly complex (Table 1). After intravenous administration there are two extremes of behavior. If $Q \ll Cl'_{int}$ and therefore extraction is high, the total drug level is relatively independent of the degree of binding in the blood, and unbound drug concentrations are simply related by f_B. On the other hand, if $Q \gg Cl'_{int}$ and hepatic extraction is low, the total drug level is inversely proportional to the free fraction, whereas binding has little effect on free concentrations. It is important that after oral administration, irrespective of the value of Cl'_{int}, total drug levels depend on binding, but free concentrations are controlled only by the intrinsic free clearance, although changes in the shape of the curve may be clearance.

Thus it may be seen that drug binding, particularly in the blood, is a critical determinant of a drug's pharmacokinetics. The various quantitative interrelationships are neither simple nor intuitive. Nevertheless, with knowledge of such factors as eliminating-organ blood flows and free intrinsic clearance, the effects of altered binding on the AUC can be reasonably well predicted. It is also apparent that characterizing a drug pharmacokinetically without considering the extent of its binding in the

TABLE 1. Relationship between the Area under the Curve (AUC) for Total and Free Drug and the Physiological Determinants of Hepatic Clearance and Route of Administration

Route of administration			AUC (total)	AUC (free)
Intravenous		General	$\dfrac{D(Q + f_B Cl'_{int})^a}{Q f_B Cl'_{int}}$	$\dfrac{D(Q + f_B Cl'_{int})}{Q Cl'_{int}}$
	$Q \ll Cl'_{int}$		$\dfrac{D}{Q}$	$\dfrac{D f_B}{Q}$
	$Q \gg Cl'_{int}$		$\dfrac{D}{f_B Cl'_{int}}$	$\dfrac{D}{Cl'_{int}}$
Oral		All cases	$\dfrac{D}{f_B Cl'_{int}}$	$\dfrac{D}{Cl'_{int}}$

[a] Q, total organ blood flow; f_B, fraction of unbound drug in blood; Cl'_{int}, free intrinsic clearance of drug from organ's intracellular water; D, dose of administered drug.

blood is insufficient if a meaningful mechanistic interpretation of changes in parameter values is to be possible.

DISPOSITION OF BENZODIAZEPINES AND AGING

Benzodiazepines are prescribed extensively in the elderly but the use of these drugs presents some therapeutic problems. The frequency of adverse reactions to diazepam, chlordiazepoxide (3), and flurazepan (14) is considerably higher in the elderly than in young patients. Such findings are consistent with the concept of an increased responsiveness of elderly patients to these drugs. However, the relative contributions of altered receptor sensitivity (5, 9, 28) versus changes in the drugs' pharmacokinetics are unclear.

The presence of age-related changes in the disposition of benzodiazepines was first demonstrated with diazepam (20). In a group of 33 normal healthy predominantly male subjects, the elimination half-life of diazepam increased linearly by about four- to fivefold from age 15 to 82 years. This prolongation from about 20 to 90 hours was independent of the cigarette smoking habits of the individuals, and the phenomenon has been confirmed by others (13, 15, 25). Interestingly, the change is not associated with a decrease in the systemic clearance of total drug; rather, diazepam distribution increases with age. This is apparent in both the initial volume into which drug distributes almost instantaneously after rapid intravenous administration (V_1) and the volume of distribution at steady state (Vd_{ss}), whether the estimates are in absolute volumes or corrected for body weight. The increases are also present if the volumes are calculated in terms of unbound drug (20, 25). Diazepam is extensively N-dealkylated, and significant plasma levels of desmethyldiazepam appear after even a single dose. With increasing age, the first appearance of this pharmacologically active metabolite is delayed; peak concentrations are lower and occur later (20). It has been demonstrated recently that systemic clearance of desmethyldiazepam is reduced in the elderly, leading to a threefold prolongation of the elimination half-life (21). However, there is apparently no statistically significant age-related increase in the distribution volume, although a trend exists.

A similar age-associated perturbation in disposition to that observed with diazepam may also occur with nitrazepam (19). Following single oral dosing, the mean elimination half-life in geriatric patients is about 40 hours compared to 30 hours in young healthy volunteers. Furthermore, the apparent oral clearance is not different between the two groups, whereas the distribution volume increases twofold. In contrast, Castleden et al. (5) were unable to find any pharmacokinetic difference between young and elderly normal subjects. The reason for this discrepancy is unclear at present, but it may be related to the use of bedridden elderly patients (23) who were also receiving multiple concurrent drug therapy. Normal relatively healthy patients might react differently.

The postdistribution elimination half-life of chlordiazepoxide is also longer in elderly normal male subjects than in their younger counterparts (30, 33). The prolongation was linearly related to age over the range 16 to 86 years, and the relative change was somewhat larger than with diazepam; a six- to sevenfold increase from about 6 hours at age 20 to about 36 hours at age 80. The peak plasma levels of desmethylchlordiazepoxide also were significantly reduced with increasing age. As with diazepam, a two- to threefold linearly correlated increase in the volume of distribution at steady state contributed to the lengthening of the half-life. In addition, however, in contrast to diazepam, there was a significant reduction in the systemic clearance of unbound and total chlordiazepoxide from about 30 to 8 ml/min over the age range 20 to 80 years.

In contrast to the aforementioned benzodiazepines, the disposition of lorazepam (12, 22) appears to be relatively unaffected by aging. Plasma levels of both unchanged drug and the conjugated metabolite, as well as the latter's urinary excretion profile, were similar in both young and elderly normal nonsmoking males from 15 to 73 years old, and no statistical correlations were present between age and any pharmacokinetic parameter (22). A confirmatory study using cross-sectional groups of young and elderly subjects has revealed a small but statistically significant increase (11%) in the distribution volume in the older group and a small decrease in systemic clearance. However, when cigarette smokers were excluded no decrease was observed (12). The disposition of oxazepam, which likewise is metabolized extensively by conjugation with glucuronic acid, also appears to be independent of age (36).

Thus, with increasing age the disposition of certain benzodiazepines changes quantitatively, but despite the close chemical and pharmacologic similarities, there does not appear to be any consistent pattern. The large increase in distribution volume is perhaps the more unusual and unexpected finding, since the known pathophysiologic changes occurring with aging would be expected to produce the opposite effect. For example, the decrease in total body water (35) and the reduction in lean body mass (27), i.e., V_T of equation (3), would produce a smaller volume of distribution. This is seen clearly with ethanol (38) and antipyrine (39). Similarly, the decrease in tissue perfusion (1) would be expected to reduce at least the initial distribution space and lengthen the time to reach pseudo-tissue equilibrium, as observed with morphine (2). Clearly, then, the augmented distribution must be caused by an increase in the ratio of f_B/f_T.

The 1,4-benzodiazepines are bound fairly extensively to plasma constituents, of which albumin is generally considered to be the most important (37). Since the serum albumin level is reduced in the elderly (11, 42), it might be predicted that the unbound drug fraction would be increased in this population, leading to greater extravascular distribution. However, the major studies from our group were unable to find any relationships between age and plasma binding for diazepam (20), chlordiazepoxide (30), lorazepam (22) and oxazepam (36). These findings have been confirmed recently using an improved technique and additional subjects (18). Other studies have failed to estimate the binding parameter with the exception of that of Macklon et al. (25) with diazepam. The Macklon study confirmed the earlier pharmacokinetic findings of Klotz et al. (20) with regard to total drug but, in addition, found a statistically significant linear reduction in diazepam plasma binding with age. Accordingly, the systemic clearance of unbound drug decreased with age; this could account for some of the increase in the distribution volume. Methodologic differences may be involved in these conflicting data. It is becoming increasingly apparent that several confounding factors may be present in the estimation of the unbound fraction, and these may be contributing to the discrepancies in the literature.

For ease and convenience, clinical disposition studies requiring frequent blood collection often use an indwelling intravenous cannula into which repeated doses of heparin are administered to maintain patency. Recent studies indicate that this procedure may affect significantly the apparent plasma binding of the benzodiazepines (6). A dose of only 100 U of heparin doubles the free fractions of diazepam, chlordiazepoxide, and oxazepam within 90 seconds, and the effect persists for about 30 to 45 minutes (Table 2). Interestingly, the binding of lorazepam is not affected. Presumably, the effect involves the release of lipase from the capillary endothelium and the liberation of fatty acids, which then displace the drugs from their plasma binding sites. It is not known whether the binding phenomenon is age dependent, but this may be likely since the free fatty acid response to heparin is reduced in the elderly (32). In any case, it is now clear that blood samples for binding and pharmacokinetic purposes should be obtained only by venipuncture or from a saline-irrigated cannula.

An increasing amount of data suggests gender may also be a factor in the

TABLE 2. Effect on the Percentage of Benzodiazepine Unbound in the Plasma in Young Normal Nonfasting Subjects Determined 90 Seconds after 100 U Intravenous Heparin

	Before heparin	After heparin
Diazepam	1.0 ± 0.2	4.4 ± 2.3[a]
Chlordiazepoxide	4.6 ± 0.6	8.7 ± 3.9[a]
Oxazepam	4.4 ± 0.5	6.3 ± 1.0[a]
Lorazepam	9.4 ± 0.9	9.9 ± 1.9

[a] $p < .05$.

disposition of some benzodiazepines (13, 15, 16), in part through sex differences in plasma binding. The elimination half-life of chlordiazepoxide is almost twice as long in young women than in men the same age, and concurrent use of oral contraceptives prolongs the value further (29). No significant differences exist in the systemic clearance of total drug, but the steady-state distribution volume is larger in women than in men, and contraceptive use increases it further (Table 3). These distribution differences apparently are due to differences in plasma binding, since estimation of the volumes in terms of unbound drug indicates no significant effects. We have observed similar sex-related differences in the plasma binding of diazepam (unpublished observation). Whether such gender-related phenomena persist throughout life is not known, but it may be significant that 27 of the 33 subjects observed by Klotz et al. (20) were men, and 12 of 19 subjects studied by Macklon et al. were women (25).

A final potential confounding factor in assessing the extent of plasma binding is a subject's possible use of other drugs, prescription and nonprescription. Even though the drugs may not be metabolic enzyme inducers or inhibitors, they may have a dispositional effect. Wallace et al. (40) found, for example, that the free plasma fraction of salicylate and sulfadiazine was significantly greater in elderly patients receiving other drugs than in those not on any drug therapy, and the effect was augmented if two or more drugs were involved.

In conclusion, therefore, the precise contribution of altered binding in the plasma/blood to the age-related increase in distribution of diazepam and chlordiazepoxide is not now well defined. However, it is significant

TABLE 3. Pharmacokinetics of Clordiazepoxide in Young Healthy Men and Women

Parameter	Males	Females not taking oral contraceptive steroids	Females taking oral contraceptive steroids
$t_{1/2}$	8.9 ± 2.5	14.8 ± 5.9[a]	24.3 ± 12.0
V_1 (l/kg)	0.18 ± 0.06	0.27 ± 0.11	0.38 ± 0.13
Vd_{ss} (l/kg)	0.33 ± 0.12	0.40 ± 0.14	0.62 ± 0.23[b]
Vd_{ss}, unbound drug (l/kg)	11.9 ± 4.9	9.2 ± 4.6	10.1 ± 4.2
Systemic clearance, total drug (ml/min/kg)	0.43 ± 0.12	0.35 ± 0.17	0.34 ± 0.12
Systemic clearance, unbound drug (ml/min/kg)	15.6 ± 5.3	8.7 ± 5.0[b]	5.7 ± 3.0
Percent plasma binding	97.0 ± 1.2	95.5 ± 1.4[b]	93.6 ± 1.5[b]

[a] $p < .05$, men versus women not taking oral contraceptives.

[b] $p < .05$, women not taking oral contraceptives versus females taking oral contraceptives.

that the augmented distribution of diazepam is still present when distribution is estimated in terms of unbound drug (20, 25). Accordingly, it must be concluded that an age-associated change in tissue binding (f_T) must occur. This parameter is poorly defined with regard to determining factors and is very difficult to estimate directly in vivo. The required increase in tissue binding might be explained intuitively by the relative increase in body fat with age, especially since the age-related changes are only seen with the more lipophilic benzodiazepines, diazepam and chlor-diazepoxide, but not with oxazepam and lorazepam. But the fact that the distributional change is observed with diazepam almost immediately after intravenous injection, when distribution to fat is minimal (26), suggests that other factors may be involved. Also, it is perhaps noteworthy that the distribution alteration is already present in the late teens and early 20s, when fat deposition is usually not apparent. Membrane permeability changes as well as intracellular macromolecule binding may be involved.

A major question resulting from the dispositional studies I have described is their significance in the enhanced cerebral responsiveness of the elderly. At present, this is difficult to answer definitively, since a number of assumptions and extrapolations are required. The ultimate effect of the benzodiazepines is thought to be by way of a specific receptor (4) that depends on the unbound neuronal drug concentration for inter-action. In turn, unbound concentration is in relatively rapid equilibrium with free blood concentration and intracellularly bound drug. Since the systemic (hepatic) clearances of the benzodiazepines in man are all less than 100 ml/min, the circulating unbound drug level is independent of binding in the blood, irrespective of the route of administration (Table 1). Thus it is unlikely that any age-related changes in f_B contribute to the age-related increase in clinical responsiveness following acute drug admin-istration. The consideration of changes in tissue binding (f_T) leads to a similar conclusion, since the resulting increase in the volume of distribu-tion causes a reduction in the unbound circulating drug level. Following chronic drug therapy, the free plasma concentration depends only on the systemic clearance of unbound drug, i.e., intrinsic free clearance. Thus an increased responsiveness in the elderly could be explained by a reduction in Cl'_{int}. This would appear to be the case with chlordiazepoxide and possibly diazepam. Such increased effective drug levels could be en-hanced further if the elimination of psychopharmacologically active metabolites is impaired with age.

CONCLUSION

Studies of drug disposition play an important role in the elucidation of altered drug responsiveness in individuals or certain populations. They are in fact essential before any assessment of altered pharmacodynamics can be made. Nevertheless, caution must always be taken in interpreting such findings. This is particularly so if perturbations in drug binding to blood constituents and tissues are involved. In these circumstances it appears essential that the disposition of unbound drug be recognized as the prime factor. Such an approach requires both an appropriate in vitro method for estimating binding and an awareness of the various factors affecting the phenomenon. Unless this information is available and appropriate steps taken in experimental design, incorrect conclusions regarding the effects of age on drug disposition may be drawn.

REFERENCES AND BIBLIOGRAPHY

1. Bender AD (1965): The effect of increasing age on the distribution of peripheral blood flow in man. J Am Geriat Soc 13:192–198.
2. Berkowitz BA, Ngai SH, Yang JC, Hempstead J, Spector S (1975): The disposition of morphine in surgical patients. Clin Pharmacol Therapeut 17:629–635.
3. Boston Collaborative Drug Surveillance Program (1973): Clinical depression of the central nervous system due to diazepam and chlordiazepoxide in relation to cigarette smoking and age. N Engl J Med 288:277–280.
4. Braestrup C, Squires RF (1978): Brain specific benzodiazepine receptors. Br J Psychiatry 133:249–260.
5. Castleden CM, George CF, Marcer D, Hallett C (1977): Increased sensitivity to nitrazepam in old age. Br Med J 1:10–12.
6. Desmond PV, Roberts RK, Wood AJJ, Dunn GW, Wilkinson GR, Schenker S (1980): Effect of heparin administration on plasma binding of benzodiazepines. Br J Clin Pharmacol 9:171–175.
7. Evans GH, Shand DG (1973): Disposition of propranolol VI. Independent variation in steady-state circulating drug concentrations and half-life as a result of plasma drug binding in man. Clin Pharmacol Therapeut 14:494–500.
8. Gibaldi M, McNamara PJ (1978): Apparent volumes of distribution and drug binding to plasma proteins and tissues. Europ J Clin Pharmacol 13:373–378.
9. Giles HG, McLeod SM, Wright JR, Sellers EM (1978): Influence of age and previous use on diazepam dosage required for endoscopy. Can Med Assoc J 118:513–514.
10. Gillette JR (1971): Factors affecting drug metabolism. Ann NY Acad Sci 179:43–66.
11. Greenblatt DJ (1979): Reduced serum albumin concentration in the elderly: A report from the Boston Collaborative Drug Surveillance Program. J Am Geriat Soc 27:20–22.
12. Greenblatt DJ, Allen MD, Locniskar A, Harmatz JS, Shader RI (1979): Lorazepam kinetics in the elderly. Clin Pharmacol Therapeut 26:103–113.
13. Greenblatt DJ, Allen MD, Harmatz, JS, Shader, RI (1979): Age, sex and diazepam kinetics. Clin Pharmacol Therapeut 27:301–312.
14. Greenblatt DJ, Allen MD, Shader RI (1977): Toxicity of high dose flurazepam in the elderly. Clin Pharmacol Therapeut 21:355–361.
15. Greenblatt DJ, Harmatz JS, Shader RI (1978): Factors influencing diazepam pharmacokinetics: Age, sex, and liver disease. Int J Clin Pharmacol 16:177–179.
16. Greenblatt DJ, Harmatz JS, Stanski DR, Shader RI, Franke K, Koch-Weser J (1977): Factors influencing blood concentrations of chlordiazepoxide: A use of multiple regression analysis. Psychopharmacology 54:277–282.
17. Hurwitz N (1969): Predisposing factors in adverse reactions to drugs. Br Med J 1: 536–539.

18. Johnson RF, Schenker S, Roberts RK, Desmond PV, Wilkinson GR (1979): Plasma binding of benzodiazepines in humans. J Pharm Sci 68:1320–1322.

19. Kangas L, Iisalo E, Kanto J, Lehtinen V, Pynnönen S, Ruikka I, Salminen J, Sillanpää M, Syvälahti E (1979): Human pharmacokinetics of nitrazepam: Effect of age and diseases. Europ J Clin Pharmacol 15:163–170.

20. Klotz U, Avant GR, Hoyumpa A, Schenker S, Wilkinson GR (1975): The effects of age and liver disease on the disposition and elimination of diazepam in man. J Clin Invest 55:347–359.

21. Klotz U, Müller-Seydlitz P (1979): Altered elimination of desmethyldiazepam in the elderly. Br J Clin Pharmacol 7:119–120.

22. Kraus JW, Desmond PV, Marshall JP, Johnson RF, Schenker S, Wilkinson GR (1978): Effects of aging and liver disease on disposition of lorazepam. Clin Pharmacol Therapeut 24:411–419.

23. Levy G (1967): Effect of bed rest on distribution and elimination of drugs. J Pharm Sci 56:928–929.

24. Yacobi, A, Levy G (1975): Comparative pharmacokinetics of common anticoagulants XIV: Relationship between protein binding, distribution, and elimination kinetics of warfarin in rats. J Pharm Sci 64:1660–1664.

25. Macklon AF, Barton M, James O, Rawlins MD (1979): The effect of age on the pharmacokinetics of diazepam. Clin Sci 59:479–583.

26. Marcucci F, Fanelli R, Frova M, Morselli PL (1968): Levels of diazepam in adipose tissue of rats, mice and man. Europ J Pharmacol 4:464–466.

27. Novack LP (1972): Aging, total body potassium, fat-free mass, and cell mass in males and females between ages 18 and 85 years. J Gerontol 27:438–443.

28. Reidenberg MM, Levy M, Warner H, Coutinho CB, Schwartz MA, Yu G, Cheripko J (1978): Relationship between diazepam dose, plasma level, age, and central nervous system depression. Clin Pharmacol Therapeut 23:371–374.

29. Roberts RK, Desmond PV, Wilkinson GR, Schenker S (1979): Disposition of chlordiazepoxide: Sex differences and effects of oral contraceptives. Clin Pharmacol Therapeut 25:826–831.

30. Roberts RK, Wilkinson GR, Branch RA, Schenker S (1978): Effect of age and parenchymal liver disease on the disposition and elimination of chlordiazepoxide (Librium). Gastroenterology 75:479–485.

31. Rowland M, Benet LZ, Graham GG (1973): Clearance concepts in pharmacokinetics. J Pharmacokin Biopharm 1:123–136.

32. Rubegni M, Bandinelli C, Provvedi D (1974): Heparin induced lipolysis in the elderly. Lancet 2:903.

33. Shader RI, Greenblatt DJ, Harmatz JS, Franke K, Koch-Weser J (1977): Absorption and disposition of chlordiazepoxide in young and elderly male volunteers. J Clin Pharmacol 17:709–718.

34. Shand DG, Cotham RH, Wilkinson GR (1976): Perfusion-limited effects of plasma drug binding on hepatic drug extraction. Life Sci 19:125–130.

35. Shock NW, Watkin DM, Yiengst BS, Norris AH, Gaffney GW, Gregerman RI, Falzone JA. (1963): Age differences in the water content of the body as related to basal oxygen consumption in males. J Gerontol 18:1–8.

36. Shull HJ, Wilkinson GR, Johnson R, Schenker S (1976): Normal disposition of oxazepam in acute viral hepatitis and cirrhosis. Ann Int Med 84:420–425.

37. van der Kleijn E (1969): Protein binding and lipophilic nature of ataractics of the meprobamate- and diazepine-group. Arch Int Pharmacodyn 179:225–250.

38. Vestal RE, McGuire EA, Tobin JD, Andres R, Norris AH, Mezey E (1977): Aging and ethanol metabolism. Clin Pharmacol Therapeut 21:343–354.

39. Vestal RE, Norris AH, Tobin JD, Cohen BH, Shock NW, Andres R (1975): Antipyrine metabolism in man: Influence of age, alcohol, caffeine and smoking. Clin Pharmacol Therapeut 18:425–432.

40. Wallace S, Whiting B, Runcie J (1976): Factors affecting drug binding in plasma of elderly patients. Br J Clin Pharmacol 3:327–330.

41. Wilkinson GR, Shand DG (1975): A physiological approach to hepatic drug clearance. Clin Pharmacol Therapeut 18:377–390.

42. Woodford-Williams E, Alvarez AS, Webster D, Landless B, Dixon MP (1964/65): Serum protein patterns in "normal" and pathological ageing. Gerontologia 10:86–99.

2

QUANTITATIVE PREDICTORS OF DRUG ENTRY INTO AND DISTRIBUTION WITHIN THE BRAIN

Stanley I. Rapoport

Many drugs that do not produce central nervous system toxicity in younger individuals do so frequently in the aged. For example, the toxicity of an average daily dose of flurazepam increases from 1.9% in subjects under age 60 years to as much as 71% in people over 80 years of age (9, 13, 39).

The greater drug toxicity in elderly individuals has been ascribed to slowed metabolism with resultant accumulation of toxic quantities in the brain, to decreased plasma-protein binding, or to a reduction in renal clearance or distribution volumes. It remains possible, however, that age-related changes in the intensity and time course of a drug effect are due to alterations in the number or sensitivity of brain receptors. Consequently, a normally tolerable brain concentration can lead to a toxic response. During aging, various changes occur in brain neuron/glia ratios, regional brain glucose consumption, dendritic arborization and spine number of brain neurons, neurotransmitter concentrations, the histology of brain tissue, overall behavior, and possibly in the blood–brain barrier (1, 15, 29, 41–43).

The blood–brain barrier at the cerebral vasculature (Figure 1) is composed of a continuous layer of endothelial cells connected by tight junctions (*zonulae occludentes*), close intercellular connections that prevent intercellular diffusion of water-soluble nonelectrolytes, ions, and proteins. Vesicular transport furthermore is minimal at the cerebrovascular endo-

From the Laboratory of Neurosciences, National Institute on Aging, Gerontology Research Center, Baltimore City Hospitals, Baltimore, Maryland.

A. Raskin, D. S. Robinson, and J. Levine, eds., Age and the Pharmacology of Psychoactive Drugs.

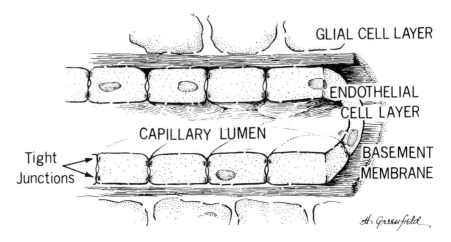

FIGURE 1. Diagram of blood–brain barrier at capillary level. (From Rapoport [31].)

thelium. Thus, the layer as a whole has properties of an extended lipoid cell membrane and is permselective for lipid-soluble as opposed to water-soluble substances (31, 37).

The selective permeability of the barrier to lipid-soluble drugs explains different rates of drug passage from plasma to spinal fluid and brain and may account for observed correlations between therapeutic effectiveness of a centrally acting drugs and lipid solubility (4). For example, the effectiveness of a centrally acting drug in a given homologous series increases with lipid solubility, as is illustrated in Figure 2 for barbiturates, hydantoins, and imides (21, 31). In Figure 2, the octanol/water partition coefficient is taken as a measure of lipid solubility (18).

Lipid-soluble agents equilibrate rapidly between brain and blood. It is not difficult therefore to estimate their brain concentrations from their plasma levels, once a steady-state brain/plasma measurement has been made in an animal model. On the other hand, the intensity and time course of a central response to a poorly permeant, less lipid-soluble drug may not be related simply to the plasma level, because of restricted blood–brain exchange and limited intracerebral distribution (10, 31, 39). For such drugs, it is important to know which factors quantitatively determine their rates of entry into the brain and their distribution within brain tissue.

This question was approached by first establishing a general relation between cerebrovascular permeability and the octanol/water partition coefficient for different substances and then by considering how drugs distribute within the brain parenchyma. The appendix at the end of this

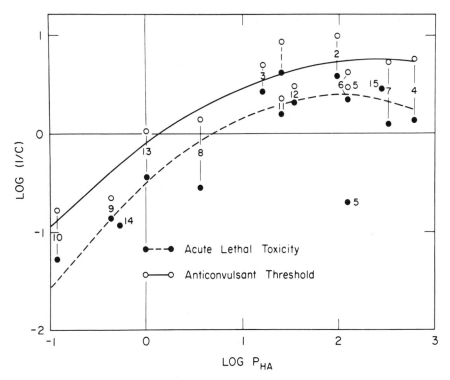

FIGURE 2. Effective threshold for anticonvulsant action and lethal toxicity of a series of barbiturates, hydantoins, and imides as related to the octanol/water partition coefficient P_{HA} of the undissociated compound. Closed circles denote toxicity, open circles anticonvulsant threshold to seizures induced in mice by pentylenetetrazol, as taken from Millichap (21). P_{HA} values and least squares curves are from Lien et al. (19), excluding point 5 for calculation of the toxicity curve. The compounds are phenobarbital (1), mephobarbital (2), metharbarbital (3), petharbarbital (4), primidone (5), mephenytoin (6), albutoin (7), phenacemide (8), trimethadione (9), dimethadione (10), phensuximide (11), methsuximide (12), ethosuximide (13), acetazolamide (14), chlordiazepoxide (15). Concentration (C), millimoles. (From Rapoport [31].)

chapter presents an extended model of blood–brain exchange that explicitly takes into account transfer at the cerebral capillary, loss of material from brain to cerebrospinal fluid, and intracellular sequestration, binding, or metabolism. In the following discussion, a simplified two-compartment model is considered that has been used to examine experimentally blood–brain barrier permeability and intracerebral drug distribution in short-term studies in conscious rats.

CURRENT METHODS OF MEASURING CEREBROVASCULAR
PERMEABILITY AND BLOOD–BRAIN EXCHANGE

Current techniques to measure cerebrovascular transfer in animal experiments are useful for substances that enter the brain rapidly, but not at a
moderate or slow rate. For example, the brain uptake index (BUI)
technique appears to show that opioid peptides do not penetrate the
blood–brain barrier (7), whereas a more sensitive compartmental analysis
method, presented later, demonstrates that these peptides penetrate the
barrier at a significant rate (33).

Excluding the method of compartmental analysis, four major techniques
are used at present to measure cerebrovascular permeability in animals—
the indicator dilution technique, the single-injection external-registration
technique, the brain uptake index technique and the concentration profile
analysis technique. These techniques were reviewed in 1976 by Rapoport
(31). With the indicator dilution technique, a diffusible test tracer is
injected together with an indiffusible reference tracer into the carotid artery
of an animal, and sagittal sinus blood is sampled periodically thereafter (8).
Extraction of the test tracer by brain is calculated from the ratio of test to
reference concentration in venous effluent. With the single-injection
external-registration technique, brain uptake is monitored externally and
continuously by a collimated scintillation detector over the skull, following
intracarotid injection of a single radioactive test tracer (30). With the brain
uptake index (BUI) technique, a test ^{14}C-tracer is injected together with a
very diffusible reference tracer (e.g., ^{3}HOH) into the carotid circulation
(3, 27). The animal is decapitated 5 to 15 seconds later, and brain
^{14}C and ^{3}H concentrations are measured and used to calculate a BUI
as follows:

$$\text{BUI} = \frac{^{14}C_{brain}/^{3}H_{brain}}{^{14}C_{injectate}/^{3}H_{injectate}} \tag{1}$$

The higher the BUI, the higher the cerebrovascular permeability of the ^{14}C
test agent. In the technique involving concentration profile analysis (28), a
tracer is infused through the cerebral ventricles of an animal until a steady-
state diffusion profile is established within the brain substance. Analysis of
the profile provides an estimate of cerebrovascular permeability.

These techniques have several limitations. None provides accurate
permeability coefficients of poorly penetrating compounds, such as peptides, L-glucose, mannitol, sucrose, or methotrexate. All apply to the brain
as a whole but not to specific brain regions. Also, all require that cerebral
blood flow be known. They are inaccurate if pathologic or altered physiologic conditions cause flow to change in specific brain regions (26, 31).

CEREBROVASCULAR PERMEABILITY AND LIPID SOLUBILITY
IN CONSCIOUS ANIMALS

The method of compartmental analysis was used to measure the cerebro-vascular permeability and cerebral distribution volume of a number of different substances in conscious rats (25, 33). Conscious rather than anesthetized animals were used to ensure consistent regional cerebral blood flows. Flow must be known in order to calculate regional cerebro-vascular permeability of lipid-soluble substances.

A radiotracer was injected as an intravenous (IV) bolus. Femoral artery radioactivity was measured and fit by the least squares method to the following equation, where C_{art} dpm/ml is the concentration of unbound tracer in plasma, A_i (dpm/ml) and α_i (sec^{-1}) are constants, t is time (seconds) and n is 3 to 4:

$$C_{art} = \sum_1^n A_i e^{-\alpha_i t} \tag{2}$$

Figure 3 illustrates a typical plasma curve following an IV injection of ^{14}C-mannitol, and gives constants for the best fit of equation (2) to the data (25).

In the absence of cerebral binding, intracellular sequestration, or brain metabolism (factors taken into account in the model presented in the Appendix), brain uptake is given as follows: C_{brain} dpm/g is parenchymal (extravascular) concentration, P cm sec^{-1} is cerebrovascular permeability, A is 240 cm^2/cm^3 (or cm^{-1}) (capillary surface area), $\bar{C}_{br\ cap}$ dpm/ml is mean concentration in cerebral capillaries, and V is cerebral distribution volume of tracer,

$$dC_{brain}/dt = PA(\bar{C}_{br\ cap} - C_{brain}/V) \tag{3}$$

$\bar{C}_{br\ cap}$ is related as follows to the measured arterial plasma concentration and measured regional cerebral blood flow F (sec^{-1})

$$\bar{C}_{br\ cap} = (F/PA)\ (C_{art} - C_{brain}/V)(1 - e^{-PA/F}) + C_{brain}/V \tag{4}$$

$\bar{C}_{br\ cap}$ approximates C_{art} if $PA \ll F$, i.e., if little tracer is extracted from the capillary, but is less than C_{art} if extraction is high because permeability is large. Substituting equation (4) into equation (3) gives, for $M = F(1 - e^{-PA/F})$,

$$dC_{brain}/dt = M(C_{art} - C_{brain}/V) \tag{5}$$

Thus, brain accumulation is proportional to the concentration difference between arterial plasma and brain multiplied by a factor M, which is less than PA to the extent that tracer is extracted during its passage through the

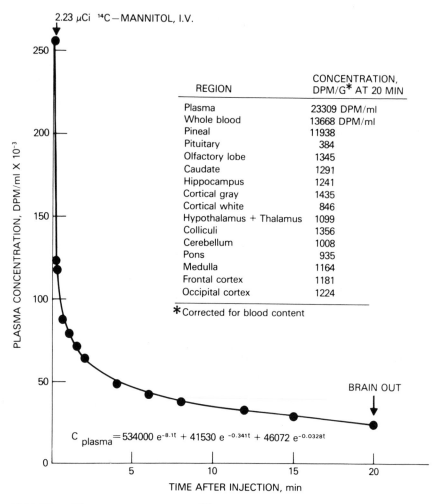

FIGURE 3. Plasma concentrations of ^{14}C-mannitol following intravenous injection and regional brain concentrations 20 minutes after injection. The curve is a fit of equation (2) to the data points, with t in minutes (From Ohno et al. [25].)

cerebral capillary. Substituting equation (2) into equation (5) and integrating to time T of decapitation gives $C_{\text{brain}}(T)$ in terms of two unknowns, M (or PA) and V:

$$C_{\text{brain}}(T) = \sum_{1}^{n} \frac{MA_i}{M/V - \alpha_i} (e^{-\alpha_i T} - e^{-MT/V}) \qquad (6)$$

PA alone can be obtained simply from experiments limited to such short times after IV injection of tracer so that $C_{\text{brain}}/V \ll C_{\text{art}}$. In this case, back diffusion from brain to plasma is negligible in equation (5), and that equation is integrated to give

$$PA = -F \ln_e \left(1 - C_{\text{brain}}(T)/F \int_0^T C_{\text{art}} dt \right) \qquad (7)$$

For poorly penetrating substances, furthermore, $C_{\text{brain}}(T)/\int_0^T C_{\text{art}} dt \approx$ 0. Equation (7) then simplifies to give PA in terms of measured brain concentration at T and the integrated arterial plasma concentration,

$$PA = C_{\text{brain}}(T)/ \int_0^T C_{\text{art}} dt \qquad (8)$$

Table 1 presents blood flows F and blood volumes in different brain regions of conscious rats (25, 26). F was used in equations (6) and (7). Intravascular radioactivity was calculated as regional blood volume (ml/g) times whole blood concentration (dpm/ml). C_{brain} was calculated as net tissue radioactivity minus intravascular radioactivity. $\int_0^T C_{\text{art}}$ was obtained when necessary, by integrating the plasma concentration curve.

Equation (6) or (7) was fit to data for different nonelectrolytes and organic electrolytes to estimate individual values of PA and V. Figure 4 illustrates that P, which was calculated by dividing PA by $A = 240$ cm^{-1}, is directly related to the octanol/water partition coefficient. The relation indicates that substances penetrate the blood–brain barrier mainly because of their lipid solubility, although deviations from the regression line show that permeability is determined as well by such factors as size, steric and electronic configuration, and interaction with cell membranes (36).

TABLE 1. Regional Cerebral Blood Volume and Blood Flow in Conscious Rats

Brain region	Blood volume (ml g^{-1} ×,100)	Blood flow (F) (sec^{-1})
Olfactory bulb	4.68 ± 0.23 (4)[a]	0.017 ± 0.0016 (6)
Caudate nucleus	1.24 ± 0.25	0.030 ± 0.0031
Hippocampus	1.61 ± 0.16	0.023 ± 0.0027
Frontal lobe	2.09 ± 0.04	0.028 ± 0.0048
Occipital lobe	2.42 ± 0.26	0.030 ± 0.0049
Thalamus + hypothalamus	1.79 ± 0.10	0.025 ± 0.0028
Superior colliculus ⎱ Inferior colliculus ⎰	2.01 ± 0.20	0.028 ± 0.0028 0.034 ± 0.0042
Cerebellum	3.46 ± 0.26	0.017 ± 0.0019
Pons	2.56 ± 0.27	0.021 ± 0.0020
Medulla	3.53 ± 0.70	0.020 ± 0.0022
Grey matter, parietal	2.70 ± 0.40	0.040 ± 0.0061
White matter	1.14 ± 0.22	0.019 ± 0.0023

Data from Refs. (25) and (26).

[a]Mean ± SEM (number of animals).

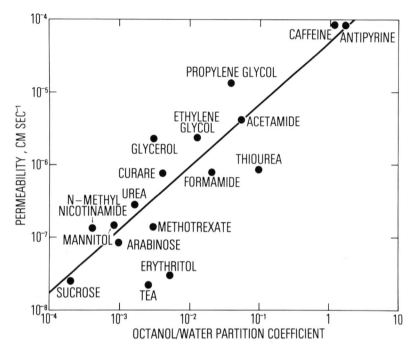

FIGURE 4. Relation between cerebrovascular permeability and octanol/water partition coefficient for different substances. (Data from Rapoport et al. [36].)

Membrane permeability should depend directly on the octanol/ water partition coefficient if transfer occurs by simple diffusion through an aporous lipoid membrane (6, 11). The relation in Figure 4, which is consistent with this theory, occurs as well at lipoid membranes of single cells. Furthermore, cerebrovascular permeability of different agents is like that at membranes of single cells and at aporous bimolecular lipid membranes. These facts suggest that intravascular drugs enter the brain by dissolving in and diffusing through lipoid endothelial cell membranes of cerebral capillaries, without passing through aqueous membrane pores or interendothelial tight junctions (25, 31, 36).

The curve-fitting procedure with equation (5) also showed that $V \approx 0.1$, when the octanol/water partition coefficient equaled 10^{-4} ($P \approx 10^{-8}$ cm sec^{-1}), $V \approx 0.4$ when the coefficient equaled 10^{-3} ($P \approx 10^{-7}$ cm sec^{-1}), and $V \approx 0.8$ when the coefficient exceeded 10^{-2} ($P \geq 10^{-6}$ cm sec^{-1}). Substances with partition coefficients above 1 were not examined but are known to accumulate in brain lipids to make V exceed 1 (20, 31). The relation between V and partition suggests that, in short-term experiments, very water-soluble agents (e.g., sucrose) enter the brain extracellular space (about 25% of brain wet weight), slightly lipid-soluble agents (e.g., glycerol) enter cells as well to some extent, and lipid-soluble agents (e.g., caffeine, antipyrine) easily cross cell membranes and distribute in all of brain water (about 80% of brain wet weight) (31). It should be noted, however, that V as calculated by equation (5) represents a single empirical volume of distribution derived from acute experiments. A more realistic approach, which also applies to steady-state experiments, takes into account solute distribution within both intracellular (or bound) and extracellular compartments, as well as loss to cerebrospinal fluid (see Appendix).

Figure 4 makes it possible, within error limits of the regression line, to predict cerebrovascular permeability P from only the partition coefficient of a given agent. For more accuracy, P and V can be measured directly by the compartmental analysis method. Once P and V are known, equation (6) can be used to relate brain uptake to the history of the plasma concentration of a drug.

Predicted uptakes are illustrated in Figure 5 for different permeabilities, following a step elevation in free plasma concentration (Figure 5a) or a bolus injection of material (Figure 5b). The figure legend shows which values of V were used in relation to permeability and partition. Equation (6) should be of use in analyzing plasma–brain exchange of drugs in man, if correct values of regional cerebral blood flow are employed (Table 1) (17).

In this analysis, C_{art} represents the plasma concentration of free drug not

FIGURE 5. Brain concentration, as predicted by equation (6), in relation to cerebrovascular permeability, following a step elevation of free plasma concentration (A) or a bolus injection (B) of substance. V was taken as 0.1 for $P = 10^{-8}$ cm sec^{-1}, as 0.4 for $P = 10^{-7}$ cm sec^{-1}, and as 0.8 for $P \geq 10^{-6}$ cm sec^{-1}. Note that Vs for steady-state analysis (equation [6]) are approximate, because they were calculated from single-injection studies. (From Rapoport et al. [36].)

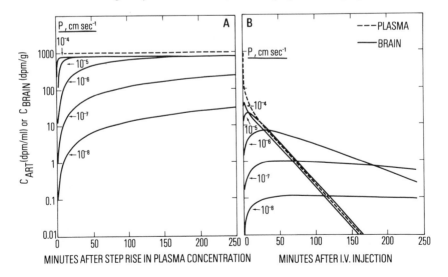

bound to protein, so that protein binding must be measured for analysis (cf. Table 2). Furthermore, the free concentration of a weak acid or base refers to the free plasma concentration of undissociated species, which is four orders of magnitude more lipid soluble than the charged, dissociated species (18). The effective partition coefficient, P^*, which determines cerebrovascular permeability of a weak acid, HA, for example, is the product of the partition coefficient of the undissociated species P_{HA} and of the plasma fraction of undissociated species, where K_a is the dissociation coefficient of HA (31):

$$P^* = P_{HA} \frac{1}{1 + 10^{pH - pK_a}} \tag{9}$$

CEREBROVASCULAR PERMEABILITY TO OPIOID PEPTIDES

With the method of compartmental analysis, it is possible to measure cerebrovascular permeabilities that cannot be characterized by the BUI method. The BUI technique was used to demonstrate that opioid peptides are impermeable at the blood–brain barrier, despite reported central effects when they are administered systemically (7, 38). With the compartmental analysis method it has been shown that four synthetic opioid peptides are as permeant at the blood–brain barrier as is glycerol, urea, or thiourea (Figure 4 and Table 2) (33).

TABLE 2. Cerebrovascular Permeability P of Four Synthetic Opioid Peptides

	[D-Ala²]-Met enkephalin amide	[D-Ala⁶²,¹⁴C-homoarg⁶⁹] β-lipotropin 61-69	[D-Ala²,¹⁴C-homoarg⁹] α-endorphin	[D-Ala²,¹⁴C-homoarg] β-endorphin
Brain region	Permeability (cm sec⁻¹ × 10⁶)			
Caudate nucleus	2.4 ±0.2[a]	1.3 ±0.5	2.1 ± 0.8	4.4 ± 2.7
Hippocampus	1.7 ± 0.4	1.2 ± 0.2	1.8 ± 0.8	3.1 ± 2.3
Thalamus plus hypothalamus	2.4 ± 0.2	1.2 ± 0.2	2.1 ± 1.0	2.7 ± 1.7
Frontal lobe	2.5 ± 0.3	1.5 ± 0.5	2.5 ± 1.1	3.5 ± 2.0
Pons	2.3 ± 0.3	1.7 ± 0.2	3.1 ± 1.3	4.0 ± 2.7
Peptide property				
Molecular weight	587	1000	1826	3436
O/W partition	0.066	0.012	0.0017	0.013
Unbound fraction in plasma	0.21	0.84	0.34	0.20

Data from Ref (33).
[a]Estimate ± SE of estimate ($n = 3$ to 8).

Figure 6 illustrates predicted brain concentrations following a step increase or IV bolus injection of one of the peptides examined, [D-Ala^2,^{14}C-homoarg^9]-α-endorphin. Equation (6) was used to generate the curves in the figure, with P and V as given in Table 2. The distribution volume 0.25 approximates the brain extracellular space. The half-time for filling this space, following a step rise in free plasma concentration, is about 6 minutes ($t_{1/2} = 0.693V/M$ in equation [6]). Significant brain concentrations can accumulate if permeability is the order of 10^{-6} cm sec^{-1}, provided the peptide remains in plasma for several minutes.

CEREBROVASCULAR INTEGRITY IN OLD RATS

The method of compartmental analysis was also used to demonstrate that cerebrovascular integrity does not decrease during senescence in the rat (35). It has been suggested, because blood concentrations of brain-reactive antibodies increase with age in man and animals, that the blood–brain

FIGURE 6. Peptide uptake by caudate nucleus as predicted by equation (6), following step concentration elevation or bolus injection. Plasma concentration represents unbound peptide, which composes 34% of the total plasma peptide. $P = 2.2 \times 10^{-6}$ cm sec^{-1} and $V = 0.25$ (Table 2). (From Rapoport et al. [33].)

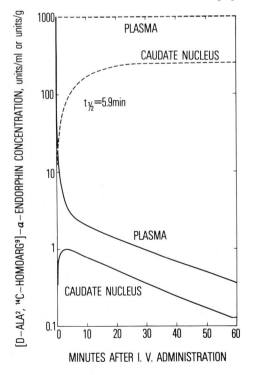

barrier breaks down during senescence, and that barrier breakdown might augment interaction between brain antigen and the peripheral immune system (22).

The hypothesis of age-related barrier damage was tested by measuring cerebrovascular permeability to ^{14}C-sucrose, in 3-month- and 28-month-old Fischer 344 rats. The permeability of sucrose normally is so low (6 $\times 10^{-8}$ cm sec^{-1}), that any alteration in barrier integrity would increase it demonstrably. Table 3 shows that cerebrovascular permeability to sucrose is not elevated in aged rats, except possibly at one region, and thus that there is no evidence of age-related breakdown of cerebrovascular integrity (34). It remains possible, however, that age-related changes occur in stereospecific transport of substrates for brain metabolism, as such changes are reported under physiologic conditions other than aging (12).

OSMOTIC OPENING OF THE BLOOD–BRAIN BARRIER

The known relations between the central effectiveness of drugs in a homologous series and lipid solubility, as illustrated for some substances in Figure 2, have stimulated efforts to synthesize lipid-soluble drugs that can easily enter the brain. In some cases, however, as with methotrexate and its esters, the lipid-soluble derivatives have not proved more effective

TABLE 3. Cerebrovascular Permeability to ^{14}C-Sucrose in 3-Month- and 28-Month-Old Fischer 344 Rats

Brain region	P (cm sec^{-1} $\times 10^8$)	
	Control rats	Aged rats
Olfactory bulb	3.10 ± 0.41^a	2.49 ± 0.22
Caudate nucleus	2.27 ± 0.12	1.87 ± 0.17
Hippocampus	2.24 ± 0.34	2.49 ± 0.21
Frontal lobe	2.98 ± 0.22	2.94 ± 0.31
Occipital lobe	2.61 ± 0.13	2.94 ± 0.11
Thalamus plus hypothalamus	2.46 ± 0.19	2.45 ± 0.18
Superior colliculus	2.75 ± 0.18	2.33 ± 0.15
Inferior colliculus	2.68 ± 0.06	2.61 ± 0.22
Cerebellum	2.73 ± 0.22	2.73 ± 0.17
Pons	2.20 ± 0.03	2.02 ± 0.11
Medulla	2.08 ± 0.04	2.17 ± 0.14
Midbrain	2.18 ± 0.12	2.18 ± 0.06
Grey matter	3.07 ± 0.25	2.92 ± 0.32
White matter	1.55 ± 0.22	2.38 ± 0.15^b
Average	2.49	2.47

Data from Ref. (35).
^{a}Mean $\pm$ SEM ($n = 3$).
^{b}Differs significantly from control mean ($p < .05$).

against brain tumors than the poorly permeable water-soluble parent compound (14). In other cases, critical brain enzymes that are genetically absent, yet might be effective when allowed into the brain, cannot be altered enough to allow them to diffuse through the blood–brain barrier (2). One possible approach to therapy of brain disease in these cases is to modify cerebrovascular permeability reversibly to allow the water-soluble parent compound into the brain.

The blood–brain barrier consists of a continuous layer of endothelial cells that are connected by tight junctions, as illustrated in Figure 1. This continuous endothelium can be opened reversibly by infusing, into the carotid circulation, a concentrated solution of arabinose or mannitol. Physiologic and ultrastructural studies indicate that hypertonic solutions shrink cerebrovascular endothelial cells and reversibly widen interendothelial tight junctions, without producing long-term pathologic or behavioral changes (31, 32).

We recently employed the osmotic method to increase brain uptake of methotrexate, a drug that is potentially useful to treat brain tumors (23, 24, 44). Table 4 demonstrates the effect of a 30-second infusion of 1.6m arabinose solution into the right carotid artery on right-sided cerebrovascular permeability to ^{3}H-methotrexate in the rat. The tracer was injected

TABLE 4. Cerebrovascular Permeability to ^{3}H-Methotrexate in Uninfused Rats or Following Right-Sided Carotid Infusion of Either Isotonic Saline or 1.6m Arabinose Solution

Brain region	Methotrexate permeability (cm sec^{-1} × 10^7)		
	Uninfused controls (3)[a]	Isotonic saline infusion (3)	1.6m arabinose infusion (3)
Olfactory bulb	2.02 ± 0.77[b]	2.61 ± 0.73	9.62 ± 2.25[c]
Caudate nucleus	1.68 ± 0.35	2.28 ± 0.50	8.42 ± 1.25[c]
Hippocampus	1.24 ± 0.41	3.01 ± 0.56	9.21 ± 0.83[c]
Frontal lobe	1.42 ± 0.35	2.03 ± 0.45	11.21 ± 1.46[c]
Occipital lobe	0.98 ± 0.33	2.00 ± 0.43	11.75 ± 1.08[c]
Thalamus plus hypothalamus	1.45 ± 0.19	2.18 ± 0.36	10.92 ± 1.67[c]
Superior colliculus	1.34 ± 0.27	1.88 ± 0.45	12.00 ± 1.83[c]
Inferior colliculus	1.56 ± 0.20	2.53 ± 0.54	7.83 ± 1.17[c]
Cerebellum	1.40 ± 0.50	1.98 ± 0.66	6.25 ± 1.50[c]
Pons	1.28 ± 0.08	1.57 ± 0.05	1.36 ± 0.16
Medulla	1.28 ± 0.43	1.02 ± 0.46	6.83 ± 1.96[c]

Data from Ref. 24.

[a]Number of animals.

[b]Mean ± SEM.

[c]Differs (p < .05) from uninfused control brains.

5 minutes after osmotic treatment, and the animal was killed 10 minutes thereafter. Permeability was calculated by equation (8).

Perfusion of the right hemisphere with isotonic saline did not significantly increase ^{3}H-MTX permeability, whereas 1.6m arabinose elevated permeability sevenfold, compared to permeability in uninfused brain. Brain uptake was augmented by an additional factor of 7 when ^{3}H-MTX was administered into the right carotid circulation rather than systemically. The combined effect of osmotic treatment followed by carotid administration of drug increased brain uptake by a factor of about 50, above levels obtained with systemic administration without osmotic infusion (23, 24).

CONCLUSION

A method of compartmental analysis is presented to study cerebrovascular permeability and distribution volume of drugs in conscious rats to predict brain uptake of systemically administered drugs from the time course of the plasma concentration. This method should help to ascertain whether an increase in drug toxicity in man with aging is related to an altered brain concentration of the drug or of its derivatives, or to altered cerebral receptor sensitivity. In conscious rats, tracers were injected as an IV bolus and their entry into the brain was analyzed in terms of a two-compartment model that provided estimates of cerebrovascular permeability and cerebral distribution volume. Permeability was roughly related to the octanol/water partition coefficient, which suggests that substances enter the brain by first dissolving in the lipoid membranes of the continuous cerebrovascular endothelium that constitutes the blood–brain barrier at cerebral capillaries. Compartmental analysis also was used to show that cerebrovascular integrity remains intact in the senescent rat, that synthetic opioid peptides have a significant cerebrovascular permeability, and that the blood–brain barrier can be made sevenfold more permeable to intravascular methotrexate, an anticancer drug, by infusing hypertonic arabinose solution into the carotid artery. The compartmental model can be extended to take into account extracellular and intracellular (or bound) disposition of drug within the brain, as well as loss from brain to cerebrospinal fluid. The extended model should be useful for studying steady-state brain/plasma drug distribution as well as brain concentrations following single dose regimens.

APPENDIX

Equation (5), which describes brain uptake of a substance in relation to permeability and a single brain distribution volume, applies best to single-dose procedures or to short-term conditions with IV infusion but is less useful for long-term experiments that approach the steady state. Furthermore, equation (5) ignores intracerebral compartmentation and loss to or uptake from cerebrospinal fluid (CSF). Some of these factors are taken into account in the following extended analysis, which should be applicable to steady-state as well as to short-term conditions.

Let plasma, brain extracellular space, and brain intracellular space (containing *either* free tracer, bound tracer, or metabolized tracer) be three compartments (designated 0, 1, and 2) with radiotracer (or chemical) concentrations equal to X_0, X_1, and X_2, respectively. Because brain specific gravity approximates 1 (31), X_0 is in units of mole/milliliter, and X_1 and X_2, in units of mole/gram.

Figure 7 is a flow diagram that represents material exchange between plasma and brain extracellular fluid, and between extracellular fluid and CSF on the one hand and an intracellular compartment (free, bound, or metabolized) on the other. (For simplicity, it is assumed that tracer is lost to CSF.) The ks are transfer constants in units of seconds^{-1}, so the following equations represent time-dependent concentration changes in brain compartments 1 and 2,

$$\dot{X}_1 = k_1 X_0 + k_4 X_2 - (k_2 + k_3 + k_5)\, X_1$$
$$\dot{X}_2 = k_3 X_1 - k_4 X_2 \tag{A-1}$$

FIGURE 7. Flow diagram for exchange between plasma, brain extracellular fluid, CSF, and intracellular or bound compartment. ks represent transfer constants (sec^{-1}), and X_0, X_1, and X_2 represent compartmental concentrations in plasma, extracellular fluid, and an intracellular (or bound) compartment, respectively.

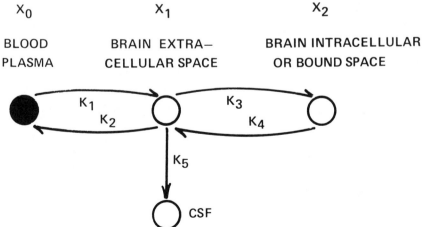

Let $k_6 = k_2 + k_3 + k_5$. Rearranging equation (A-1) gives, with the operational notation $D = d/dt$,

$$(D + k_6)X_1 - k_4X_2 = k_1X_0$$
$$-k_3X_1 + (D + k_4)X_2 = 0$$

(A-2)

Elimination of X_2 gives the following, where $k_7 = k_4 + k_6$ and $k_8 = k_4 \times (k_2 + k_5)$:

$$(D^2 + k_7D + k_8)X_1 = k_1(D + k_4)X_0$$

(A-3)

The two roots of the homogeneous equation are λ_1 and λ_2, so

$$\lambda_1 = \frac{k_7 + \sqrt{k_7^2 - 4k_8}}{2} \quad \text{and} \quad \lambda_2 = \frac{k_7 - \sqrt{k_7^2 - 4k_8}}{2}$$

(A-4)

So

$$(D + \lambda_1)(D + \lambda_2)X_1 = k_1(D + k_4)X_0$$

(A-5)

For the present discussion, we will consider two plasma concentration curves: (1) following a bolus injection in which terms decline exponentially and (2) following a step elevation to a constant concentration. Both conditions can be represented as (see equation [2])

$$X_0 = \sum_{1}^{n} A_i e^{-\alpha_i t}$$

(A-6)

where for a bolus injection $\alpha_i > 0$ and for a step elevation $\alpha_1 = 0$ and $n = 1$. Substituting the expression for X_0 into equation (A-5) and solving gives the general solution for X_1, where c_1 and c_2 are constants:

$$X_1 = c_1 e^{-\lambda_1 t} + c_2 e^{-\lambda_2 t} + \sum_{1}^{n} \frac{k_1(k_4 - \alpha_i) A_i e^{-\alpha_i t}}{(\lambda_1 - \alpha_i)(\lambda_2 - \alpha_i)}$$

(A-7)

Substituting the expression for X_1 (equation [A-7]) into equation (A-2) (bottom) and solving gives

$$X_2 = k_3 \left[\frac{c_1 e^{-\lambda_1 t}}{k_4 - \lambda_1} + \frac{c_2 e^{-\lambda_2 t}}{k_4 - \lambda_2} + \sum_{1}^{n} \frac{k_1 A_i e^{-\alpha_i t}}{(\lambda_1 - \alpha_i)(\lambda_2 - \alpha_i)} \right]$$

(A-8)

The initial conditions at $t = 0$ are that $X_1 = X_2 = 0$. This allows us to evaluate c_1 and c_2:

$$c_1 = \sum_1^n \frac{(\lambda_1 - k_4) k_1 A_i}{(\lambda_2 - \lambda_1)(\lambda_1 - \alpha_i)}$$

$$c_2 = \sum_1^n \frac{(k_4 - \lambda_2) k_1 A_i}{(\lambda_2 - \lambda_1)(\lambda_2 - \alpha_i)} \tag{A-9}$$

In the presence of intracellular retention or binding, the total brain concentration at any time, $X_1 + X_2$, equals the sum of the expressions in Equations (A-7) and (A-8):

$$C_{brain} = c_1 e^{-\lambda_1 t}\left(1 + \frac{k_3}{k_4 - \lambda_1}\right) + c_2 e^{-\lambda_2 t}\left(1 + \frac{k_3}{k_4 - \lambda_2}\right)$$

$$+ \sum_1^n \frac{k_1(k_4 - \alpha_i + k_3) A_i e^{-\alpha_i t}}{(\lambda_1 - \alpha_i)(\lambda_2 - \alpha_i)} \tag{A-10}$$

If the steady state is approached ($t \rightarrow \infty$), $C_{brain} \rightarrow 0$ after a bolus injection. After a step elevation in plasma concentration to $A_1(n = 1)$, however, C_{brain}/C_{plasma} approaches the following steady-state ratio [note that $\lambda_1 \lambda_2 = k_4(k_2 + k_5)$, equal to the operational steady state distribution volume $V_{t=\infty}$:

$$\frac{C_{brain}}{C_{plasma}} = \frac{k_1}{k_2 + k_5} \frac{k_3 + k_4}{k_4} = V_{t=\infty} \tag{A-11}$$

REFERENCES AND BIBLIOGRAPHY

1. Ball MJ (1978): Topographic distribution of neurofibrillary tangles and granulovacuolar degeneration in hippocampal cortex of aging and demented patients. Acta Neuropathol, 42:73–80.

2. Barranger JA, Rapoport SI, Fredericks WR, Pentchev PG, MacDermot KD, Steusing JK, Brady RO (1979): Modification of the blood-brain barrier: Increased concentration and fate of enzymes entering the brain. Proc Natl Acad Sci USA 76:481–485.

3. Bradbury MWB, Patlak CS, Oldendorf WH (1975): Analysis of brain uptake and loss of radiotracers after intracarotid injection. Am J Physiol 229:1110–1115.

4. Brodie BB, Kurz H, Schanker LS (1960): The importance of dissociation constant and lipid solubility in influencing the passage of drugs into cerebrospinal fluid. J Pharmacol Exp Ther 130:20–25.

5. Cheng DK (1959): Analysis of Linear Systems. Reading, Addison-Wesley.

6. Collander R (1937): The permeability of plant protoplasts to nonelectrolytes. Trans Faraday Soc 33:985–990.

7. Cornford EM, Braun LD, Crane PD, Oldendorf WH (1978): Blood-brain barrier restriction of peptides and the low uptake of enkephalins. Endocrinology 103:1297–1303.

8. Crone C (1963): The permeability of capillaries in various organs as determined by use of the "indicator diffusion" method. Acta Physiol Scand 58:292–305.

9. Davis JM (1975): In Fields WS, ed: Neurological and Sensory Disorders of the Elderly, New York, Stratton Intercontinental, pp 151–164.

10. Davis, JM, Erickson S, Dekirmenjian H (1978): Plasma levels of antipsychotic drugs and clinical response. In Lipton MA, DiMascio A, Killam KF, eds: Psychopharmacology: A Generation of Progress. New York, Raven Press, pp 905–915.

11. Davson H, Danielli JF (1943): The Permeability of Natural Membranes. London, Cambridge University Press, pp 80–117.

12. Gjedde A, Crone C (1975): Induction processes in blood–brain transfer of ketone bodies during starvation. Am J Physiol. 229:1165–1169.

13. Greenblatt DJ, Allen MD, Shader RI (1977): Toxicity of high-dose fluorazepam in the elderly. Clin Pharmacol Therapeut 21:355–361.

14. Johns DG, Farquhar D, Wolpert MK, Chabner BA, Loo TL (1973): Dialkylesters of methotrexate and 3',5'-dichloromethotrexate synthesis and interaction with aldehyde oxidase and dihydrofolate reductase. Drug Metab Dispos 1:580–589.

15. London ED, Nespor S, Moore L, Mahone P, Rapoport SI (1979): Age-dependent changes in local cerebral glucose utilization. Age 2:131.

16. Knott GD, Schrager RI (1972): On-line modeling by curve fitting. In Computer Graphics: Proceedings of the SIGGRAPH Computers in Medicine Symposium, 6. ACM: SIGGRAPH Notices, no. 4, pp 138–151.

17. Lassen NA, Ingvar DH, Skinhøj E (1978): Brain function and blood flow. Sci Am October, pp 62–71.

18. Leo A, Hansch C, Elkins D (1971): Partition coefficients and their uses. Chem Rev 71:525–616.

19. Lien EJ, Tong GL, Chou JT, Lien LL (1973): Structural requirements for centrally acting drugs. J Pharm Sci 62:246–250.

20. Lovell S, Dugdale AE (1973): The selection of antibodies for the initial treatment of bacterial meningitis. Med J Austal 1:529–532.

21. Millichap JG (1963): Anticonvulsant drugs. In Root WS, Hofmann FG, eds: Physiological Pharmacology, vol. 2. New York, Academic Press, pp 97–173.

22. Nandy K (1975): Significance of brain-reactive antibodies in serum of aged mice. J Gerontol 30:412–416.

23. Neuwelt EA, Maravilla KR, Frenkel EP, Rapoport SI, Hill SA, Barnett PA (1979): Osmotic blood-brain barrier disruption: Computerized tomographic monitoring of chemothera-peutic agent delivery. J Clin Invest 64:684–688.

24. Ohno K, Fredericks WR, Rapoport SI (1979): Osmotic opening of the blood-brain barrier to methotrexate in the rat. Surg Neurol 12:323–328.

25. Ohno K, Pettigrew KD, Rapoport SI (1978): Lower limits of cerebrovascular permeability to nonelectrolytes in the conscious rat. Am J Physiol 235:H299–H307.

26. Ohno K, Pettigrew KD, Rapoport SI (1979): Local cerebral blood flow in the conscious rat, as measured with ^{14}C-antipyrine, ^{14}C-iodoantipyrine and ^{3}H-nicotine. Stroke 10: 62–67.

27. Oldendorf WH (1971): Brain uptake of radiolabled amino acids, amines and hexoses after arterial injection. Am J Physiol 221:1629–1639.

28. Patlak CS, Fenstermacher JD (1975): Measurements of dog blood-brain transfer constants by ventriculocisternal perfusion. Am J Physiol 229:877–884.

29. Puri SK, Volicer L (1977): Effect of aging on cyclic AMP levels and adenylate cyclase and phosphodiesterase activities in the rat corpus striatum. Mech Ageing Dev 6:53–58.

30. Raichle ME, Eichling JO, Straatmann MG, Welch MJ, Larson KB, Ter-Pogossian MM (1976): Blood–brain barrier permeability of ^{11}C-labeled alcohols and ^{15}O-labeled water. Am J Physiol 230:543–552.

31. Rapoport SI (1976): Blood–Brain Barrier in Physiology and Medicine. New York, Raven Press.

32. Rapoport SI, Hori M, Klatzo I (1972): Testing of a hypothesis for osmotic opening of the blood–brain barrier. Am J Physiol 223:323–331.

33. Rapoport SI, Klee WA, Pettigrew KD, Ohno K (1980): Entry of opioid peptides into the central nervous system. Science 207:84–86.

34. Rapoport SI, Ohno K, Fredericks WR, Pettigrew KD (1978): Regional cerebrovascular permeability to ^{14}C-sucrose after osmotic opening of the blood–brain barrier. Brain Res 150:653–657.

35. Rapoport, SI, Ohno K, Pettigrew KD (1979): Blood–brain barrier permeability in senescent rats. J Gerontol 34:162–169.

36. Rapoport SI, Ohno K, Pettigrew KD (1979): Drug entry into the brain. Brain Res 172: 354–359, 1979.

37. Reese TS, Karnovsky MJ (1967): Fine structural localization of a blood–brain barrier to exogenous peroxidase. J Cell Biol 34:207–217.

38. Roemer D, Buescher HH, Hill RC, Pless J, Bauer W, Cardinaux F, Closse A, Hauser D, Huguenin R (1977): A synthetic enkephalin analogue with prolonged parenteral and oral analgesic activity. Nature 268:547–549.

39. Salzman C, Shader RI, Harmatz JS (1975): In Gershon S, Raskin A, eds: Aging, vol 2. New York, Raven Press, pp 259–272.

40. Scheibel ME, Lindsay RD, Tomiyasu U, Scheibel AB (1975): Progressive dendrite changes in aging human cortex Exp Neurol 47:392–403.

41. Smith CB, Fredericks WR, Rapoport SI, Sokoloff L (1979): Effects of aging on regional cerebral glucose consumption in the rat. Abstr 10th Ann Meeting Soc Neurochem Trans Amer Soc Neurochem. 10:171.

42. Tomlinson BE (1972): In Van Praag HM, Klaverboer AK, eds: Aging and the Central Nervous System. New York, De Ervon F. Bohn, pp 38–57.

43. Vernadakis A (1975): Neuronal–glial interactions during development and aging. Fed Proc 34:39–95.

44. Whiteside JA, Philips FS, Dargeon HW, Burchenal JH (1958): Intraethecal amethopterin in neurological manifestations of leukemia. Arch Intern Med 101:279–285.

3

INFLUENCE OF AGING
ON BIOGENIC AMINE SYNTHESIS:
ROLE OF THE HYDROXYLASE COFACTOR

R. A. Levine, D. M. Kuhn,
A. C. Williams, and W. Lovenberg

Interest in aging processes has led to numerous investigations concerning the relationship between alterations in neural and humoral function and increasing age. In studying the mammalian central nervous system (CNS), age-related changes in the metabolism of certain neurotransmitters, including the biogenic amines, have been described in an effort to ascertain any fundamental influences of chemical neurotransmission on aging processes. Of particular interest are human postmortem brain studies that have indicated that aspects of catecholaminergic neurotransmission are affected by increasing age in the normal population. For instance, the activity of tyrosine hydroxylase, the initial enzyme in catecholamine biosynthesis, has been shown to decline with increasing age in the human corpus striatum (15). In another study, dopamine levels were also shown to be correlated inversely with age in the striatum (3), although this finding was not confirmed in another experiment (18). These findings may have relevance to the etiology of Parkinson's disease, where there is a loss of nigrostriatal dopaminergic neurons, perhaps secondary to a premature or accelerated aging process (1). A more complete knowledge of neurotransmitter metabolism may yield greater insight into how basic regulatory mechanisms for neurotransmitter availability either contribute to or are altered by the process of aging.

In addition to Parkinson's disease, other neurologic and psychiatric disorders of the CNS are thought to involve disturbances in the metabolism of the biogenic amine neurotransmitters, particularly dopamine,

From the Section on Biochemical Pharmacology National Heart, Lung, and Blood Institute, National Institutes of Health, Bethesda, Maryland.

A. Raskin, D. S. Robinson, and J. Levine, eds., Age and the Pharmacology of Psychoactive Drugs.

norepinephrine, and serotonin. To maximize our ability to treat effectively disorders thought to involve unusual biogenic amine metabolism, it is important to understand what factors are operating in vivo to regulate the availability of these neurotransmitters at their synapses in the CNS. This chapter focuses first on the involvement of the hydroxylase cofactor, tetrahydrobiopterin, in regulating biogenic amine synthesis and, second, on the implications of studies from our laboratory relating cerebrospinal fluid (CSF) hydroxylase cofactor content to age.

BIOGENIC AMINE SYNTHESIS

In catecholaminergic neurons, neurotransmitter synthesis (Figure 1) is initiated by tyrosine hydroxylase, which catalyzes the conversion of tyrosine to dihydroxyphenylalanine (DOPA), which is decarboxylated subsequently by aromatic-L-amino acid decarboxylase to form dopamine, the final product in dopaminergic neurons. Noradrenergic neurons also are equipped with dopamine-β-hydroxylase (DBH), which catalyzes the conversion of dopamine to norepinephrine. In adrenergic neurons of the CNS and chromaffin cells of the adrenal medulla, norepinephrine is transformed into epinephrine by phenylethanolamine-N-methyltransferase (PNMT). In most instances, the activity of the initial tyrosine hydroxylase reaction regulates the rate of catecholamine biosynthesis.

FIGURE 1. Biogenic amine synthesis.

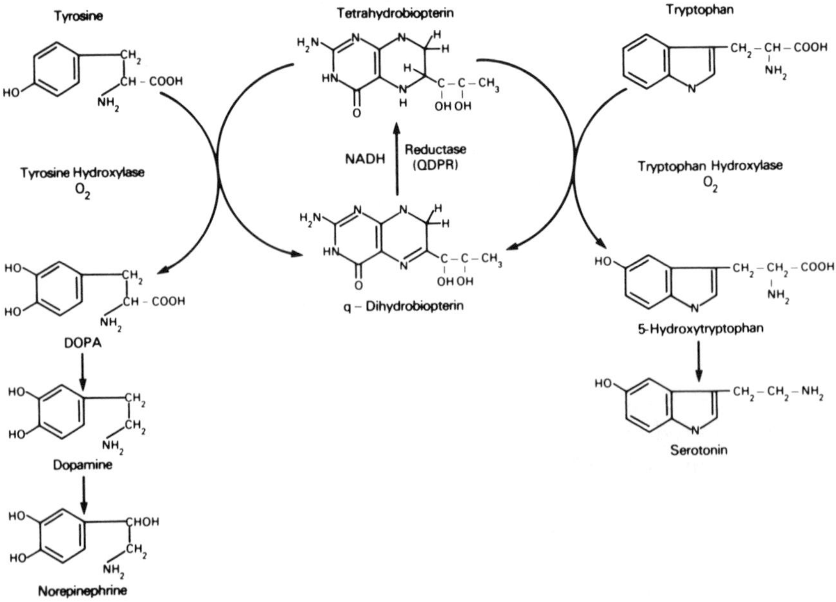

In serotonergic neurons, tryptophan is taken up and hydroxylated to 5-hydroxytryptophan (5-HTP) by tryptophan hydroxylase. Aromatic-L-amino acid decarboxylase then converts 5-HTP to 5-hydroxytryptamine (5-HT or serotonin). As in catecholamine biosynthesis, the initial hydroxylation reaction by tryptophan hydroxylase is rate limiting in serotonin synthesis. Therefore, the rate of amine biosynthesis should be coupled closely to the activities of these enzymes. An understanding of the kinetic parameters of these initial rate-limiting hydroxylase reactions is important to discover ways of manipulating in vivo enzyme activity.

INVOLVEMENT OF TETRAHYDROBIOPTERIN IN REGULATING BIOGENIC AMINE SYNTHESIS

Tyrosine and tryptophan hydroxylase are distinct mixed-function oxidase enzymes that require as cosubstrates the appropriate amino acid, molecular oxygen, and a pteridine compound in its reduced form. This pteridine cofactor is most likely tetrahydrobiopterin (also referred to as hydroxylase cofactor or BH_4). In these hydroxylation reactions (Figure 1), one atom of oxygen from O_2 is incorporated into the amino acid substrate, and BH_4 is oxidized. The oxidative product of BH_4 is the quinoid form of dihydrobiopterin (q-BH_2). The tetrahydro form, BH_4, is regenerated from q-BH_2 by quinoid dihydropterin reductase (QDPR), which uses nicotinamide adenine dinucleotide (NADH) or nicotinamide adenine dinucleotide phosphate (NADPH) as the electron donor. This reducing system is responsible for the recycling of q-BH_2 to BH_4, which is necessary for continued hydroxylation.

A variety of techniques have been employed to examine the in vivo velocities of tyrosine and tryptophan hydroxylase in both whole brain and more discrete brain areas. Estimations of in vivo activity can be compared to the maximal in vitro activities of these enzymes; comparisons of this sort have revealed that the in vivo velocities of tyrosine (13) and tryptophan (11) hydroxylase are substantially lower than their respective in vitro maximum velocities. Assuming the in vitro experiments are accurate indicators of the catalytic potential of these enzymes in vivo, it would appear that active regulatory processes are limiting their in vivo activities. Therefore, from a physiologic standpoint, these enzymes can be considered capable of achieving a much higher level of activity in order to elevate amine biosynthesis under appropriate conditions.

Tissue extracts of the corpus striatum containing high amounts of tyrosine hydroxylase in the dopamine terminals have been used for kinetic studies. The Michaelis constant (K_m) has been determined for each of the cosubstrates (O_2, tyrosine, and the cofactor, BH_4) in the tyrosine hydroxylase reaction. The K_m value of a substrate is determined by analyzing the reaction rate at varying substrate concentrations, while the other cosubstrates are present in optimal concentrations. The K_m value is an index of the affinity of a particular substrate for a particular enzyme under a standardized reaction condition. In practical terms, the K_m is the substrate concentration that will support a reaction rate equal to one-half the maximal velocity. Therefore, if prevailing substrate concentrations are at or below their K_m value, the rate of the reaction is essentially proportional to the concentration of the limiting cosubstrate in the tissue. This subsaturation of the enzyme by a cosubstrate could effectively limit the rate of tyrosine hydroxylation in vivo and therefore restrict catecholamine production. It appears that under normal conditions the in vivo concentrations of oxygen and tyrosine (2) are above their in vitro K_m values and are at or near saturation of tyrosine hydroxylase. However, the concentration of BH_4 in various brain areas appears to be well below its in vitro K_m value, and therefore its apparent subsaturation in vivo may contribute to the overall regulation of tyrosine hydroxylase (12). Similar kinetic studies have been done with tryptophan hydroxylase isolated from the mesencephalic tegmentum of the rat brain. This brain area contains a high concentration of the serotonergic cell bodies that comprise specific raphe nuclei. With regard to tryptophan hydroxylase, tryptophan concentrations are very close to K_m, so fluctuations in tryptophan levels may influence endogenous enzyme activity (4). The concentration of BH_4 in the serotonergic cell bodies also appears to be less than required for saturation (11). Consequently, BH_4 may play an important regulatory role in limiting both serotonin and catecholamine production. It should be pointed out that comparisons of this sort must be viewed with some degree of caution, because it is impossible to know the exact concentrations of cosubstrates within the aminergic neuron which is the actual site of catalysis.

Experiments in vivo have contributed to our understanding of the potential role of BH_4 in regulating catecholamine synthesis and these studies also suggest that BH_4 levels are subsaturating for tyrosine hydroxylase. Kettler and coworkers (8) injected BH_4 (30 to 1000 μg) into the cerebral ventricles of rats and reported a fourfold increase in striatal BH_4 as well as a two and one-half-fold increase in striatal catecholamine synthesis. Presumably, the increased striatal BH_4 content was elevating tyrosine hydroxylase activity, since the increase in catecholamine synthesis could be blocked by an inhibitor of tyrosine hydroxylase, α-methyl-p-tyrosine (8). Studies by Patrick and Barchas (16) also lend support to the idea that BH_4 concentrations are subsaturating for tyrosine hydroxylase in vivo. In their experiments, incubation of striatal synaptosomes in the presence of an optimal concentration (0.1 mM) of the synthetic cofactor, 6-methyl-tetrahydropterin, significantly increased synaptosomal dopamine synthesis over control levels. Conversely, Sherman and Gal (17) recently presented data that apparently demonstrate a lack of dependence of biogenic amine synthesis on the cerebral level of BH_4. Three hours after intraventricular injection of an inhibitor of BH_4 synthesis, cerebral levels of BH_4 and BH_2 were reduced by greater than 50%, while no significant reduction in dopamine, norepinephrine, or serotonin content was observed. These authors hypothesized that the rate of reduction of q-BH_2 to BH_4 by quinoid dihydropterin reductase is more important than the absolute level of cofactor in regulating biogenic amine production. However, their data did indicate a consistent decreasing trend over time in the content of all three amines (though not statistically significant). It is possible that examination of amine content longer than 3 hours after injection would reveal significantly depleted levels. In addition, these investigators made no attempt to rule out possible compensatory mechanisms, such as a kinetic activation of tyrosine or tryptophan hydroxylase, which might be operating to maintain amine production in the face of declining brain cofactor content. Analogous experiments using more discrete, predominantly aminergic brain areas are necessary to address this important question further.

Experiments in this laboratory (9) have provided indirect supportive evidence that tissue BH_4 content is important in regulating the activities of tyrosine and tryptophan hydroxylase. Studies on the regional distribution in rat brain of hydroxylase cofactor and tyrosine and tryptophan hydroxylase revealed that cofactor content was significantly correlated with both tryptophan hydroxylase and tyrosine hydroxylase and most highly correlated with total hydroxylase enzyme activity (tyrosine hydroxylase plus tryptophan hydroxylase). Consequently, cofactor content is highest in brain areas expressing high tyrosine (striatum) and tryptophan (tegmentum) hydroxylase activity and lowest in areas expressing minimal hydroxylase enzyme activity (cortex). This is consistent with the concept that BH_4 in brain is located primarily within aminergic neurons and its primary function in brain is to serve as the hydroxylase cofactor. Therefore, areas of the brain containing relatively more aminergic neurons and expressing higher hydroxylase enzyme activity would require higher cofactor content to support a greater level of amine production, assuming that the kinetic properties of each of the hydroxylase enzymes (with respect to cofactor) are similar throughout the brain.

Tetrahydrobiopterin also has an important involvement in a number of other mechanisms thought to regulate tyrosine hydroxylase activity in vitro and are also likely to occur in vivo. Tyrosine hydroxylase is subject to end-product inhibition by compounds retaining the catechol structure, of which dopamine is probably most important (12). The nature of this feedback inhibition by dopamine and other catechols is competitive with BH_4 for tyrosine hydroxylase. Thus, for any given kinetic state of tyrosine hydroxylase, catecholamine production will depend on the ratio of intraneuronal cofactor to catechol content. Theoretically, an elevation of intraneuronal BH_4 would favor the cofactor–enzyme interactions and catecholamine production could be elevated to a higher steady-state level.

The kinetic state of tyrosine hydroxylase can be altered by various treatments of the enzyme in vitro. The exposure of soluble tyrosine hydroxylase to phosphorylating conditions (ATP, cAMP, Mg^{++}, and purified cAMP-dependent protein kinase if necessary) results in a kinetic activation of the enzyme by increasing its affinity for cofactor (lower K_m) and, at the same time, decreasing the affinity of the enzyme for the major end-product inhibitor dopamine. It is presumed that this activation is accomplished by a direct phosphorylation of tyrosine hydroxylase (5). Therefore, in its phosphorylated state in vivo, tyrosine hydroxylase could use the apparent subsaturating amounts of cofactor more efficiently while being less susceptible to feedback inhibition by dopamine and other catechols. These types of regulatory mechanisms, which all involve the hydroxylase cofactor, can allow for dynamic short-term regulation of catecholamine biosynthesis by controlling the activity of existing tyrosine hydroxylase molecules.

AGE-RELATED CHANGES IN THE HYDROXYLASE COFACTOR CONTENT OF HUMAN CEREBROSPINAL FLUID

The important contributory role of BH_4 in regulating biogenic amine synthesis led our laboratory to examine hydroxylase cofactor content in human CSF, because levels may be a reflection of central aminergic function. This concept is supported by the findings that CSF cofactor content is reduced significantly in patients with Parkinson's disease and that CSF cofactor is highly correlated with CSF levels of homovanillic acid, the major metabolite of dopamine (10, 14). An altered level of CSF cofactor might be indicative of any one or more of the following: (1) a primary abnormality within the cofactor's metabolic machinery that would affect amine synthesis, (2) a compensatory altered activity state of certain central aminergic neurons in response to influences of other neuro-transmitter systems; or (3) a difference in the actual number of central aminergic neurons. In Parkinson's disease, the decreased CSF cofactor content most likely reflects the pathologic loss of nigrostriatal dopaminergic neurons. However, it is possible that altered BH_4 synthesis may play a causative role, i.e., a reduction in the synthesis of BH_4 could lead to a decrease in dopamine synthesis, "disuse" atrophy of dopaminergic neurons, and eventually, clinical parkinsonism. In fact, defects in cofactor metabolism have been demonstrated in two variant forms of phenyl-ketonuria (PKU). The elevated serum phenylalanine levels exhibited in classical PKU are caused by a defect in phenylalanine hydroxylase, the BH_4-dependent enzyme that hydroxylates phenylalanine to form tyrosine in the liver. In one variant form of PKU (7), the inability of the liver to hydroxylate phenylalanine is caused by a lack of quinoid dihydropterin reductase, the enzyme necessary for the conversion of q-BH$_2$ to BH$_4$. The other variant of PKU (6) involves a defect in liver synthesis of biopterin, restricting phenylalanine hydroxylation. It is possible that similar mechanisms are occurring in the CNS of certain patients with Parkinson's disease. Regardless, the pharmacologic elevation of brain BH$_4$ levels to increase tyrosine hydroxylase activity and dopamine production might prove to be a beneficial therapy for alleviating the clinical symptoms of Parkinson's disease.

The decreased CSF cofactor content in Parkinson's disease led us to examine the influence of age on CSF cofactor in both normal controls and parkinsonian patients. Figure 2 demonstrates that the cofactor level in normal individuals exhibits a significant ($p < .01$) decline with age. Values decreased approximately 33% over a 40-year interval from a mean of 24

FIGURE 2. CSF hydroxylase cofactor levels as a function of age in the normal subjects. (From Ref. [19].)

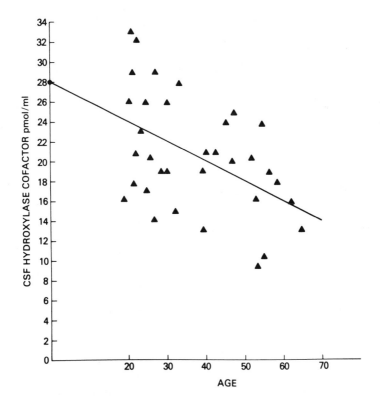

pmol/ml at age 20 to a mean of 16 pmol/ml at age 60. Patients with Parkinson's disease also exhibit a significant ($p < .01$) decline in CSF cofactor content with age as shown in Figure 3. At age 20, their estimated mean was 16 pmol/ml, which decreased to 9 pmol/ml at age 60.

This decline in CSF cofactor content with age is noteworthy because it corroborates postmortem studies demonstrating a decrease with age in dopamine content (3), tyrosine hydroxylase activity, and the number of dopaminergic neurons (15) within the human nigrostriatal system. A recent report (18) that failed to demonstrate a significant decline in dopamine content with age in the postmortem striatum casts some doubt as to whether dopamine levels are actually decreasing in the striatum. These conflicting results are indicative of the inherent difficulties with postmortem studies in general. The analysis of human CSF also has associated problems, particularly that CSF from the lumbar sac is far removed from the brain and, therefore, CSF cofactor content is, at best, an indirect indicator of central aminergic function. Nevertheless, it would appear that CSF cofactor levels reflect this apparent diminution of

FIGURE 3. CSF hydroxylase cofactor levels as a function of age in the parkinsonian patients. (From Ref. [19].)

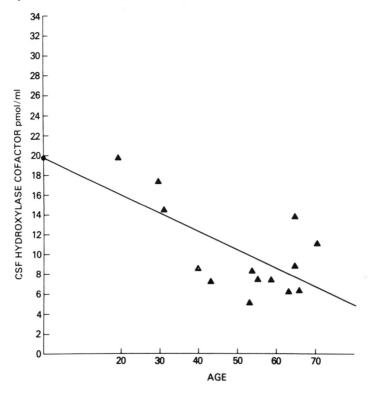

aminergic function with age and could serve as an in vivo marker for investigating these changes. If a decrease in CSF cofactor is indicative of primarily nigrostriatal dopaminergic cell loss, it may be possible through serial CSF sampling in individual patients over an extended length of time to ascertain whether there is an accelerated rate of loss of dopaminergic function contributing to the pathogenesis of Parkinson's disease. An accelerated rate in the decline of CSF cofactor with increasing age in parkinsonism would imply an active pathologic process rather than a normal aging process superimposed on a previously acquired abnormal loss of nigrostriatal neurons.

CONCLUSION

It would appear that intracellular concentrations of hydroxylase cofactor have an important regulatory role in the synthesis of the catecholamines and serotonin. This in turn may affect the functional activity of neurons using these transmitters. A procedure to measure hydroxylase cofactor in human CSF has recently been devised with the idea that this may reflect levels of cofactor within aminergic cells or the number of such cells. We have found an inverse correlation of CSF cofactor content with age. This is consistent with the known decrease in aminergic activity that occurs with aging and suggests that pharmacologic manipulation of cofactor levels in brain may have clinical significance.

REFERENCES AND BIBLIOGRAPHY

1. Barbeau A (1976): Parkinson's disease: Etiological considerations. In Yahr MD, ed: The Basal Ganglia. New York, Raven Press, pp 281–292.

2. Carlsson A, Lindqvist M (1978): Dependence of 5-HT and catecholamine synthesis on concentrations of precursor amino-acids in rat brain. Arch Pharmacol 303:157–164.

3. Carlsson A, Winblad B (1976): Influence of age and time interval between death and autopsy on dopamine and 3-methoxytyramine levels in human basal ganglia. J Neural Transm 38:271–276.

4. Fernstrom JD, Wurtman RJ (1971): Brain serotonin content: Physiological dependence on plasma tryptophan levels. Science 173:149–152.

5. Joh TH, Park DH, Reis DJ (1978): Direct phosphorylation of brain tyrosine hydroxylase by cyclic AMP-dependent protein kinase: Mechanism of enzyme activation. Proc Natl Acad Sci USA 75:4744–4748.

6. Kaufman S, Berlow S, Summer G, Milstien S, Schulman J, Orloff S, Spielberg S, Pueschel S (1978): Hyperphenylalanemia due to a deficiency of biopterin. N Engl J Med 299: 673–679.

7. Kaufman S, Holtzman NA, Milstien S, Butler I, Krumholz A (1975): Phenylketonuria due to a deficiency of dihydropteridine reductase. N Engl J Med 293:785–790.

8. Kettler R, Bartholini G, Pletscher A (1974): In vivo enhancement of tyrosine hydroxylation in rat striatum by tetrahydrobiopterin. Nature 249:476–478.

9. Levine RA, Kuhn DM, Lovenberg W (1979): The regional distribution of hydroxylase cofactor in rat brain. J Neurochem 32:1575–1578.

10. Levine RA, Williams AC, Robinson DS, Calne DB, Lovenberg W (1979): Analysis of hydroxylase cofactor activity in the cerebrospinal fluid of patients with Parkinson's disease. In Poirier LJ, Sourkes TL, Bédard PJ, eds: Advances in Neurology, New York, Raven Press, pp 303–307.

11. Lovenberg W (1977): The enzymology of tryptophan hydroxylase. In Usdin E, Weiner N, Youdim M, eds: Structure and Function of Monoamine Enzymes. New York, Marcel Dekker, pp 43–58.

12. Lovenberg W, Ames MM, Lerner P (1978): Mechanisms of short-term regulation of tyrosine hydroxylase. In Lipton MA, DiMascio A, Killam KF, eds: Psychopharmacology: A Generation of Progress, New York, Raven Press, pp 247–259.

13. Lovenberg W, Bruckwick EA (1975): Mechanisms of receptor mediated regulation of catecholamine synthesis in brain. In Usdin E, Bunny WE: Pre- and Postsynaptic Receptors. New York, Marcel Dekker, pp 149–169.

14. Lovenberg W, Levine RA, Robinson DR, Ebert M, Williams AC, Calne DB (1979): Hydroxylase cofactor activity in cerebrospinal fluid of normal subjects and patients with Parkinson's disease. Science, 204:624–626.

15. McGeer PL, McGeer EG, Suzuki JS (1977): Aging and extrapyramidal function. Arch Neurol 34:33–35.

16. Patrick RL, Barchas JD (1976): Dopamine synthesis in rat brain striatal synaptosomes. II. Dibutyryl cyclic adenosine 3' : 5'-monophosphoric acid and 6-methyltetrahydropterine-induced synthesis increases without an increase in endogenous dopamine release. J Pharm Exp Thererapeut 197:97–104.

17. Sherman AD, Gal EM (1979): Lack of dependence of amine or prostaglandin bio-synthesis or absolute cerebral level of pteridine cofactor. Life Sciences 23:1675–1680.

18. Spokes EGS (1979): An analysis of factors influencing measurements of dopamine, noradrenaline, glutamate decarboxylase and choline acetylase in human post-mortem brain tissue. Brain 102:333–346.

19. Williams AC, Ballenger J, Levine RA, Lovenberg W, Calne DB (1980): Aging and CSF hydroxylase cofactor. Neurology 30:1244–1246.

4

ONTOGENY OF THE BIOCHEMICAL BASIS FOR NEUROTRANSMISSION: IMPLICATONS FOR NEUROPSYCHOTROPIC DRUG ACTION

Joseph T. Coyle and Michael V. Johnston

Current hypotheses about the mechanisms of neuropsychotropic drug action have been developed primarily from studies of the behavioral, biochemical, and neurophysiologic effects of drugs in intact adult experimental animals. Human studies indicate, however, that many drugs have rather nonspecific effects, such as sedation in healthy individuals (16); thus, their selective therapeutic action most likely involves correction of neuronal dysfunction or its sequelae not operative under normal conditions. Interpretations of neuropsychotropic drug mechanisms in children or in the aged based on preclinical studies in adult experimental animals pose additional hazards, because at the extremes of age the neurochemical economy and functional neuronal relationships may deviate significantly from those occurring in the steady state of the mature nervous system. Indeed, clinical experience has revealed many instances of psychiatric symptom complexes and drug responses that appear unique to either childhood or late life (1, 7). Consequently, to clarify the possible age-dependent effects of psychotropic drugs, it is essential to understand the shifting neuronal substratum on which these drugs act. This chapter focuses on the development of neuronal systems in the neocortex known to interact with psychotropic drugs and on the effects of selective lesions

From the Department of Pharmacology and Experimental Therapeutics and the Department of Psychiatry and the Behavioral Sciences, Johns Hopkins University School of Medicine, Baltimore, Maryland.

Some of the research developed in this article was supported by grants from the USPHS (MH-26654) and from the National Foundation. Joseph T. Coyle is the recipient of a Research Scientist Development Award Type II, K03-00125; Michael V. Johnston has a Fellowship (NINCDS-06054).

on their ontogenetic relationships. These studies may serve as a frame-work for speculation about why neuropsychotropic drugs should have unique efects on the neurologic and behavioral disorders of childhood.

MECHANISM OF PSYCHOTROPIC DRUG ACTION

A valid generalization that can be abstracted from the last two decades of psychopharmacologic research is that the therapeutic effects and side effects of psychotropic medications result from their selective modification of chemical neurotransmission in the brain (2). To appreciate the possible sites of action of the drugs, it is helpful to review the processes involved in chemical neurotransmission. The neuron can be divided into three func-tionally distinct components: the dendrites, short projections from the cell body enriched in receptors and invested with synaptic terminals from afferent neurons; the cell body, which contains the nucleus and the protein synthetic machinery; and the axon, which extends and ramifies to make synaptic contacts with other neurons. Although the transmittal of informa-tion within a neuron from its dendrites to its axonal terminals occurs by means of a wave of electrochemical depolarization, communication between neurons occurs almost exclusively by the process of chemical neurotransmission. With a few noteworthy exceptions, neurons appear to use one chemical neurotransmitter exclusively. The neurotransmitter used by the neuron both serves as its means of communication and confers a biochemical identity on the neuron. Accordingly, the neuron contains the biochemical machinery required for the synthesis, storage, release, and inactivation of its neurotransmitter; conversely, the neuron does not usually possess the capabilities for synthesizing, storing, releasing, or inactivating neurotransmitters other than the one used. In many cases these processes are localized so highly to specific neuronal types as to constitute biochemical "markers" for them.

What are the critical biochemical processes involved in chemical neuro-transmission? Neurotransmitters are generally synthesized from neuro-physiologically inactive precursors; these substances are taken up within the nerve terminal and converted by enzymes to the neurotransmitter (Figure 1). The neurotransmitter is then concentrated and stored within vesicles in the terminal so that adequate amounts of neurotransmitter are available for release on demand. In most cases, the nerve terminals possess a high-affinity transport process on their external membrane that takes up neurotransmitter released in the synaptic cleft and thus terminates its activity. At the synapse, the area of attachment between the nerve terminal and the adjacent neuronal dendrite, highly specific receptors are con-centrated on the dendritic membrane that translate the message contained in the neurotransmitter. Activation of these receptors ultimately affects the rate of firing of the postsynaptic neurons. It is becoming apparent that

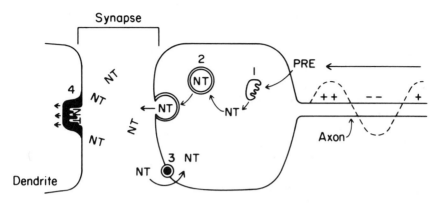

FIGURE 1. Biochemical processes mediating neurotransmission. The nerve terminal contains the biochemical machinery required to (1) synthesize, (2) store, and (3) take-up the neurotransmitter (NT) used by the neuron. Receptors (4) concentrated on the dendrites of the adjacent neuron in the area of the synapse translate the chemical message. Neurotransmitters are synthesized by specialized enzymes (1) from neurophysiologically inactive precursors (PRE). When the depolarizing action potential reaches the axon terminal, the vesicles containing neurotransmitter discharge their contents into the synaptic cleft to activate the receptors; the action of the neurotransmitter is usually terminated by reuptake (3) into the nerve terminal.

multiple types of receptors, each with its own characteristic response, exist for individual neurotransmitters; for example, norepinephrine may activate alpha-1, alpha-2, or beta-2 receptors. Ultimately it is the intensity and duration of receptor activation that determines the influence of a particular neurotransmitter system in the brain.

Psychotropic drugs exert their effects by altering one or more of these processes that either enhance or reduce the rate of neurotransmitter receptor activation. Drug effects can occur at any of the strategic sites involved in the disposition of the neurotransmitter. For example, noradrenergic neurotransmission can be enhanced by (1) increasing the availability of its precursor tyrosine, (2) releasing norepinephrine from the storage vesicles with amphetamine, (3) by inhibiting the reuptake inactivation process with tricyclic antidepressants, or (4) directly stimulating specific norepinephine receptors (e.g., alpha-2 receptor with clonidine). Conversely, noradrenergic neurotransmission can be attenuated by (1) inhibiting the synthesis of norepinephrine with alpha-methylparatyrosine, (2) depleting the storage vesicles with reserpine, or (3) directly blocking specific norepinephrine receptors (e.g., beta receptors with propranolol).

Although psychotropic drugs alter the synaptic action of specific neurotransmitters, the neuronal system affected by a particular drug does not act in a vacuum. Pathologic states reflect a disturbance in the balance among a variety of neuronal pathways innervating a particular brain region. Thus, the therapeutic effects of psychotropic drugs must be understood in terms of how the drug alters the influence of a particular neuronal system with reference to the contravailing inputs that use other types of neuro-transmitters. In considering psychotropic drug action at the extremes of age, one must take into account both the maturational differences in the critical biochemical processes on which the drug acts and the possible differences in the functional integrity of the other types of synaptic input involved in the pathologic process.

DEVELOPMENTAL SYNAPTIC CHEMISTRY OF THE CORTEX

Critical Events in Neuronal Maturation

Studies of brain development have revealed important periods in the neuronal cell life (11). First, there is the "birth" of the neuron. Neurons that form a particular brain nucleus or make up a particular cortical layer undergo a brief but intense period of mitotic activity and then cease dividing; brainstem regions are formed first, with cortical regions estab-lished later and more gradually. After the terminal mitotic event, the neurons migrate to their final resting place, whereupon they undergo differentiation.

Differentiation involves both the elaboration of dendritic and axonal processes and the appearance of the biochemical machinery required for the synthesis, storage, release, and inactivation of the neurotransmitter used by the neuron. The final stage of differentiation involves formation of synaptic relationships with the appropriate neurons in the central nervous system. Although the establishment of the neuronal circuitry of the adult brain is considered the end stage of maturation, a more subtle and gradual reformation of synapses occurs in the mature brain as adaptations are made in response to synaptic use (10).

Finally, senescence appears to have differential effects on the bio-chemical processes involved in neurotransmission, and certain neuronal populations may undergo degeneration at differing rates.

Cortical Pathways

To exemplify the importance of the principles just outlined, results from studies on the maturation of the pre- and postsynaptic processes involved in neurotransmission for three defined cortical inputs are reviewed. The cerebral cortex has been chosen since this is a likely site of action for psychotropic drugs. The three neuronal systems examined, the noradren-ergic afferents, the cholinergic afferents, and the GABAergic intrinsic neurons, have been implicated as the sites of primary therapeutic action or of side effects for several psychotropic medications (Table 1).

TABLE 1. Psychotropic Drug Interactions with Cortical Neurons

Neuronal type	Potentiate	Attenuate
Noradrenergic	Tricyclic antidepressants Stimulants Monoamine oxidase inhibitors Alpha agonists (clonidine)	Reserpine Beta-blockers
Cholinergic	Physostigmine Precursors (choline, lecithin)	Atropinelike drugs
GABAergic	Benzodiazepines Barbiturate anticonvulsants	Convulsants (picrotoxin bicuculline)

The noradrenergic innervation to the cerebral cortex arises from cell bodies located in the locus coeruleus, a nucleus situated bilaterally in the pons under the fourth ventricle (Figure 2). Noradrenergic input is highly divergent, spreading in an anterior-to-posterior fashion to innervate all layers of the cerebral cortex (18, 20). A considerable portion of the cholinergic innervation to the cerebral cortex is derived from a group of cell bodies located in the nucleus basalis in the ventral globus pallidus (15). The cholinergic innervation to the cerebral cortex, in contrast to the

FIGURE 2. Localization of neuronal cell bodies providing cortical innervation. The distribution of GABAergic, cholinergic, and noradrenergic neurons innervating the cerebral cortex of the rat are schematically presented. LC, locus coeruleus; CC, corpus callosum; NB, nucleus basalis; Ach, acetylcholine; NE, norepinephrine.

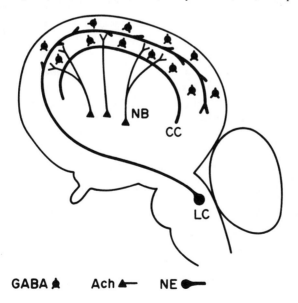

noradrenergic input, follows a radial distribution (24). The GABAergic innervation to cerebral cortex is derived primarily, if not exclusively, from stellate neurons intrinsic to the region, which are distributed uniformly throughout all layers of the cerebral cortex (21).

In these studies, the neurochemical differentiation of the neurons or their axonal terminals were monitored in the lateral cortex of the rat from birth through to adulthood. Three presynaptic markers were examined: the activity of the synthetic enzyme for the neurotransmitter, the concentration of the neurotransmitter, and the activity of the high-affinity uptake process for the neurotransmitter in isolated nerve terminal fractions (synaptosomes). Each of these parameters is highly restricted to the neurons that use the particular neurotransmitter, and each plays an important role in neurotransmission. In addition, the receptors that mediate the postsynaptic effects of the neurotransmitter were also measured by ligand-binding techniques. Taken together, these parameters provide a variation of density biochemical profile of the maturation of the component processes required for neurotransmission for each neuronal type.

Cortical Noradrenergic Innervation

In rats, the cells that form the locus coeruleus undergo a brief period of mitosis between 11 and 13 days of gestation (17). By 15 days of gestation, when the cerebral cortex is in the earliest stages of its formation, axonal processes from the nascent noradrenergic neurons invade the primordial telencephalon (3). At birth, the specific activity of tyrosine hydroxylase, the initial and rate-limiting enzyme in the synthesis pathway for norepinephrine, has attained 40% of the adult level (13) (Figure 3). Similarly, the concentration of endogenous norepinephrine and the activity of the synaptosomal uptake process for norepinephrine, an index of noradrenergic terminal density, are also approximately 40% of adult levels. Although noradrenergic terminals make up less than 1% of the total population of synapses in the adult lateral cortex, electron microscopic studies suggest that this input is one of the earliest subcortical projections to reach the cortex and contributes nearly 30% of all synaptic terminals in the neonatal cortex (5). Whereas the apparent concentration of noradrenergic terminals as measured by synaptosomal uptake of norepinephrine remains constant for the first 2 weeks after birth and then increases to approximate adult levels by 5 weeks, the specific activity of tyrosine hydroxylase and the concentration of endogenous norepinephrine exhibit a much more gradual maturation. This disparity may mean that the development of the presynaptic machinery responsible for the availability of neurotransmitters lags behind the formation of axons and terminals.

In spite of the precocious development of the noradrenergic synaptic input to the neocortex, beta-receptors, as measured by the ligand binding

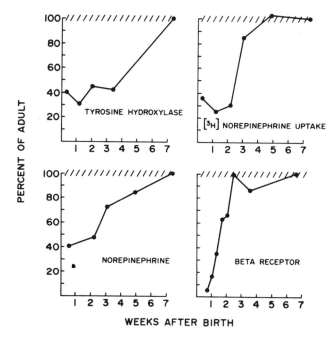

FIGURE 3. Development of the neurochemical markers for noradrenergic innervation to the cerebral cortex of the rat. The specific activities of tyrosine hydroxylase and of the synaptosomal uptake process for [³H] norepinephrine and the concentrations of norepinephrine were assayed in the developing lateral cortex of the rat. Values for beta receptor, which was measured by the specific binding of [¹²⁵I] hydroxybenzilpindolol, were taken from Harden et al. (8). Results are presented in terms of percent of the specific activity or concentration found in adult (180 g) rats. Each point is the mean of five or more separate assays from two or more litters.

techniques or by the stimulation of beta-sensitive adenylate cyclase, are virtually undetectable at birth (8). These receptors appear at approximately 5 days after birth and then exhibit a rapid increase to attain adult concentration by 12 days. Thus the noradrenergic system provides an example of a neuronal pathway that develops well in advance of one of the receptor sites that mediate its postsynaptic effects.

Cortical Cholinergic Innervation

The development of the cholinergic innervation to the lateral cortex, which arises primarily from the nucleus basalis in the globus pallidus, differs from the noradrenergic afferent system. From birth up to 10 days after birth, the levels of two presynaptic markers for the cholinergic neurons, choline acetyltransferase activity and the synaptosomal high affinity uptake process for choline remain extremely low to virtually undetectable in the lateral cortex (Figure 4). However, commencing at 10 days after birth there is a precipitous increase in these markers, which attain 50 to 60% of the adult level by 17 days after birth. These results suggest that the cholinergic innervation to the neocortex has a markedly delayed development in contrast to the noradrenergic input. However, measurement of the levels of endogenous acetylcholine provide a different perspective. The concentration of acetylcholine in the neonatal neocortex is 40% of adult levels; after a slight fall, it rises to adult concentrations between 3 and 5 weeks after birth. Thus, in the early postpartum period, there is a disproportionately high concentration of the neurotransmitter, compared to the other presynaptic markers for this neuronal system. While the reason for this disparity remains unclear, it may be that the turnover of acetylcholine is quite slow in the immature cortex, resulting in high steady-state levels (6); alternatively, it is possible that acetylcholine is

FIGURE 4. Development of the neurochemical markers for cholinergic innervation to the cerebral cortex of the rat. The specific activities of choline acetyltransferase and of the synaptosomal uptake process for [³H]choline and the concentrations of norepinephrine and of muscarinic receptor as measured by the specific binding of [³H]quinuclidinyl benzilate were assayed in the developing lateral cortex of the rat. Results are presented in terms of percent of the specific activity or concentration found in adult (180 g) rats. Each point is the mean of five or more separate assays from two or more litters.

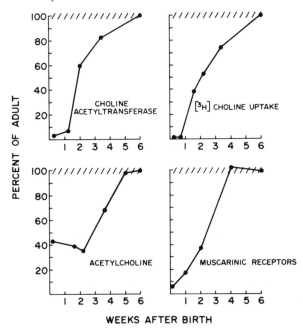

contained in noncholinergic cell types in the immature brain, since its synthesis in embryonal tissues such as the placenta has been well documented (22). Nevertheless, the muscarinic receptor, the primary acetylcholine receptor in the neocortex, exhibits a developmental profile that correlates closely with the ontogenetic changes in the specific activities of choline acetyltransferase and of the synaptosomal high-affinity uptake process for choline (6).

Cortical GABAergic Innervation

The GABAergic neurons, being intrinsic to the cerebral cortex, undergo mitosis during the last 6 days of gestation in the rat, when the neurons forming the various layers of the cerebral cortex multiply (23). The activity of glutamate decarboxylase, the enzyme that synthesizes gamma-aminobutyric acid (GABA), is quite low at birth but exhibits a steady increase in specific activity to achieve adult levels by 3 weeks after birth (Figure 5). As in the case of acetylcholine, the concentration of endogenous GABA is disproportionately high in the neonatal cortex in comparison to the specific activity of its biosynthetic enzyme. The levels of GABA increase by 2 weeks after birth to adult concentrations, where it remains thereafter. In contrast to these two presynaptic markers, the synaptosomal high-affinity uptake for GABA develops rapidly to surpass the adult specific activity by 2 weeks after birth; for the subsequent 3 weeks, it remains at 130% of adult specific activity before returning to the adult level at 7 weeks. Thus, with regard to the GABAergic system, the disparities in the developmental relationships among the presynaptic processes mediating neurotransmission result in a disproportionately greater influence of the mechanism that inactivates the synaptic action of the neurotransmitter. In spite of the high concentration of GABA in the neonatal cortex, the receptor sites that mediate its action show a delayed maturation that commences 1 week after birth (4).

Implications for Psychotropic Drug Action

Since psychotropic drugs exert their effects by altering the efficacy of synaptic neurotransmission, it is instructive to examine how the biochemical substratum on which these drugs act may differ in immature and adult rat cortexes.

With regard to the cortical GABAergic system, marked differences between 7-day olds and adults can be observed in the rate of development of the presynaptic processes that regulate the availability of GABA at the synapse and in the postsynaptic receptors. In the 7-day old, the specific activity of glutamate decarboxylase is only 15% that of adults, the concentration of GABA is 65% of adults, and the high-affinity uptake process

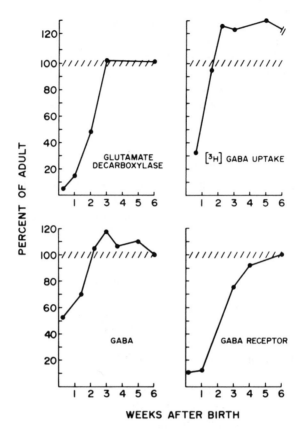

WEEKS AFTER BIRTH

FIGURE 5. Development of the neurochemical markers for GABAergic innervation to the cerebral cortex of the rat. The specific activities of glutamate
decarboxylase and of the synaptosomal uptake process for [³H] GABA and the
concentrations of GABA and of GABA receptors as measured by the specific
sodium independent binding of [³H] GABA were assayed in the developing lateral
cortex of the rat. Results are presented in terms of percent of the specific activity or
concentration found in the adult (180 g) rat. Each point is the mean of five or more
separate assays from two or more litters.

that terminates GABAs synaptic action is 60% of adults; nevertheless, the
postsynaptic receptors for GABA are only 10% of the adult level. Thus,
drugs that exert their effects by altering GABAergic neurotransmission at
either pre- or postsynaptic sites face an entirely different equation of
balance among the GABAergic processes mediating neurotransmission in
7 day olds than in adults. In altering the synaptic efficacy of a particular
neuronal system, psychotropic drugs modify the balance among the
various inputs to a brain region. The differential rates of development of
the three neuronal systems in the neocortex indicate that at various stages
of cortical maturation the relative influence of one system may differ

considerably from that occurring in the adult neocortex. Thus, at 7 days of age, the early innervation of the rat neocortex by the noradrenergic system suggests that its influence and, as a result, the effects of adrenergic drugs may be disproportionately greater than in the adult.

EFFECTS OF CORTICAL LESIONS ON THE SYNAPTIC NEUROCHEMISTRY OF THE DEVELOPING CORTEX

Prenatal Cortical Lesions

Although developmental studies shed light on the normal process of biochemical differentiation of cortical inputs, they do not address the issue of the effects of brain damage on cortical neurochemical maturation. To explore this issue, we have taken advantage of the fact that dividing cells are uniquely vulnerable to treatments that interfere with DNA synthesis (9, 23).

A potent alkylating agent with a brief half-life, methylazoxymethanol acetate, was administered to pregnant rats at 15 days of gestation (Figure 6). At this time, the neuroblasts forming the intermediate layers of the cerebral cortex are undergoing mitosis, whereas the neurons in the deep

FIGURE 6. Mechanism of cytotoxicity of methylazoxymethanol acetate. After intraperitoneal injection, methylazoxymethanol is converted rapidly to the highly reactive intermediate, diazomethane, which covalently binds to purine bases in nucleic acids. Cells in the process of synthesizing DNA for division are uniquely vulnerable and degenerate. In contrast, cells that are postmitotic and differentiating or cells that are not actively dividing but will undergo mitosis in the future (G_0 phase) are relatively insensitive.

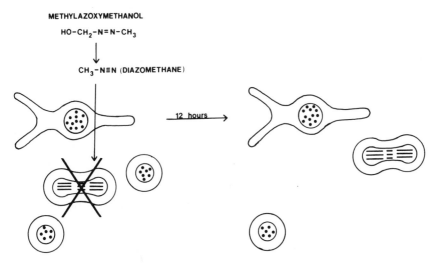

layers of cerebral cortex, as well as the cholinergic perikarya in the nucleus basalis and the noradrenergic perikarya in the locus coeruleus, have ceased dividing and commenced differentiation. Treatment with methyl-azoxymethanol at this time results in a selective ablation of the neurons that form the intermediate layers of the neocortex, while sparing the subcortical cholinergic and noradrenergic inputs (12). Fetal exposure to the drug reduces the weight of the lateral neocortex in adulthood by nearly 70% owing to the selective loss of neurons located in cortical layers II, III, and IV; however, the weight and appearance of the brainstem and cerebellum remain virtually normal. Although the lesion is quite severe, it resembles damage produced by a variety of fetal insults in man.

The presynaptic markers (neurotransmitter synthesizing enzyme, endogenous neurotransmitter, and synaptosomal uptake process for the neurotransmitter) and postsynaptic receptors were measured throughout postnatal development in the lesioned neocortex and compared to age-matched controls (Table 2). Since the GABAergic neurons are evenly distributed throughout all layers of the lateral neocortex, the ablation of

TABLE 2. Effects of Fetal Methylazoxymethanol Lesion on Cortical Synaptic Chemistry

	3 days old	Adult
	Percent of age-matched controls	
Cortical weight	61^a	35^a
GABAergic		
Glutamate decarboxylase	114	87
GABA	108	102
[^{3}H]GABA uptake	100	106
Noradrenergic		
Tyrosine hydroxylase	295^a	314^a
Norepinephrine	240^a	242^a
[^{3}H]Norepinephrine uptake	243^a	270^a
Cholinergic		
Choline acetyltransferase	115	221^a
Acetylcholine	101	196^a
[^{3}H]Choline uptake	100^b	190^a

Pregnant rats at 15 days of gestation received either methylazoxymethanol acetate (MAM 20 mg/kg) or an equal volume of diluent by intraperitoneal injection. Offspring were killed at 3 days after birth or in adulthood (>6 weeks after birth) and their lateral cortices were dissected according to white matter landmarks. Values are presented in terms of concentration of neurotransmitters or specific activities of enzyme and synaptosomal transport processes in the MAM treated rats as compared to diluent treated rats; at least five rats in each group from at least two litters were assayed. (From Ref [13].)

$^a p < .01$ by Student's t-test.

^{b}[^{3}H]choline uptake is detectable at 3 days of age.

intermediate layers should not result in an alteration in the concentration of cortical GABAergic markers. Consistent with this assumption, virtually no differences in the concentration of the presynaptic markers for the GABAergic neurons were detected between the lesioned cortexes and controls at any point during postnatal development, although the total amount of GABAergic markers in the lateral cortex was reduced by approximately 70%.

In other words, the deficits in the GABAergic markers were commensurate with the reduction in cortical mass. In contrast, the concentration of the presynaptic markers for the noradrenergic terminals innervating the lesioned lateral cortex were consistently and significantly elevated by at least 100% in the atrophic cortex. Nevertheless, the total amount of the presynaptic markers in the lesioned cortex did not differ remarkably from those in control at the various stages of postnatal maturation. Hence, the biochemical results suggest that the noradrenergic terminal arbor developed normally but was compressed within this smaller volume of the atrophic lateral cortex. This interpretation was confirmed by immunocytochemical studies of noradrenergic fiber distribution with antisera to dopamine-beta-hydroxylase, the final enzyme in the synthesis pathway for norepinephrine (14). In the atrophic cortex, the noradrenergic axons were markedly increased in density; notably, the laminar-specific pattern of their distribution was quite disrupted (19).

The response of cholinergic innervation of the neocortex to the developmentally incurred lesion differed from that of both the noradrenergic and GABAergic systems. Until 10 days after birth, the concentration of presynaptic markers in the lesioned neocortex was similar to that in control; however, the cholinergic markers subsequently increased dramatically in concentration, ultimately surpassing control levels by nearly 60%. Although the absolute concentration of cholinergic markers nearly doubled in the atrophic adult cortex, the total amount of cholinergic markers was decreased significantly compared to control.

Implications of Fetal Brain Damage on Psychotropic Drug Action

The effects of fetally induced neocortex lesions on the development of defined cortical inputs demonstrate that pathologic alterations in synaptic relationships observed in adulthood are not fixed throughout postnatal development. The effects of the lesion must be considered both in the context of the changing pattern of synaptic relationships during maturation and with regard to possible transneuronal influences that may affect neuronal differentiation (11). Selective ablation of the neurons that form the intermediate layers of the lateral cortex at 15 days of gestation have markedly different effects on the differentiation of the GABAergic, cholinergic, and noradrenergic neurons in the cortex. If it can be assumed that the concentration of presynaptic markers for a neurotransmitter system correlates in some fashion with the degree of influence of the neuronal pathway, these lesion studies would suggest that the relative influence of GABAergic neurons is unaffected, that of the noradrenergic afferents is increased consistently throughout development, whereas the cholinergic system is unaffected initially but is increased during the later stages of maturation. Thus, the equation of balance among neuronal systems altered by psychotropic drugs differ not only in the lesioned cortex in adulthood but may also be quite different from both normal and the adult situation at earlier stages of development. These factors clearly may affect the mode of action of neuropsychotropic drugs administered at different stages of brain maturation.

CONCLUSION

The biochemical processes that mediate synaptic neurotransmission are the substrate on which psychotropic drugs exert their effects. In considering psychotropic drug action at the extremes of age, one must appreciate that the relative levels of these biochemical processes may deviate significantly from those occurring in the mature brain. In examining the postnatal development of three defined neuronal systems in the lateral cortex, several maturational variables were identified that may affect psychotropic drug action.

First, the presynaptic mechanisms responsible for the disposition of neurotransmitter (synthetic enzymes, endogenous stores of neurotransmitter, and high affinity inactivation uptake) do not develop in synchrony; as a result, the equation of balance among these processes may be different in the immature neuron than in the fully differentiated neuron.

Second, since psychotropic drugs ultimately alter the level of activation of neurotransmitter receptors, it is important to note that the receptors may develop independently of the presynaptic processes mediating neurotransmission.

Third, psychotropic drugs modify the synaptic efficacy of a particular neurotransmitter relative to other inputs. Thus, the shifting balance among the developing neuronal systems, which mature at different rates, may result transiently in relationships that deviate considerably from those in the adult brain. Finally, brain damage occurring during development may considerably alter the pattern of relationships among the surviving neurons; in effect, the pathologic sequelae of the lesion in adulthood provides an imperfect profile of the altered but shifting synaptic relationships in the maturing brain. As a consequence, theories concerning psychotropic drug action derived from studies done in normal adult experimental animals can be applied to the brain at extremes of age only with considerable caution.

We thank Carol Kenyon and Victoria Rhodes for secretarial assistance.

REFERENCES AND BIBLIOGRAPHY

1. Campbell M (1978): Use of drug treatment in infantile autism and childhood schizophrenia. In Lipton MA, DiMascio A, Killam KF, eds: Psychopharmacology: A Generation of Progress, New York, Raven Press, pp 1451–1461.

2. Cooper JR, Bloom FE, Roth RH (eds) (1978): The Biochemical Basis of Neuropharmacology, Ed 3. New York, Oxford University Press.

3. Coyle JT (1977): Biochemical aspects of neurotransmission in the developing brain. Int Rev Neurobiol 20:65–103.

4. Coyle JT, Enna SJ (1976): Neurochemical aspects of the ontogenesis of GABAergic neurons in the rat brain. Brain Res 111:119–133.

5. Coyle JT, Molliver ME (1977): Major innervation of newborn rat cortex by monoaminergic neurons. Science 196:444–447.

6. Coyle JT, Yamamura HI (1976): Neurochemical aspects of the ontogenesis of cholinergic neurons in the rat brain. Brain Res 118:429–440.

7. Eisdorfer C, Fann W (eds): (1973): Psychopharmacology and Aging. New York, Plenum Press.

8. Harden TK, Wolfe BB, Sporn JR, Perkins JP, Mollinoff PB (1977): Ontogeny of beta-adrenergic receptors in rat cerebral cortex. Brain Res 125:99–108.

9. Hicks SP, D'Amato CJ, Lowe MJ (1959): The development of the mammalian nervous system I. Malformation of the brain, especially cerebral cortex induced in rats by radiation. J Comp Neurol 113:435–469.

10. Horn G, Rose SPR, Batison PPG (1973): Experience and plasticity in the central nervous system. Science 181:506–514.

11. Jacobson M (ed)(1978): Developmental Neurobiology, ed. 22. New York, Plenum Press.

12. Johnston MV, Coyle JT (1979): Histological and neurochemical effects of treatment with methylazoxymethanol on rat neocortex in adulthood. Brain Res 170:135–155.

13. Johnston MV, Coyle JT (1980): Ontogeny of neurochemical markers for noradrenergic, GABAergic and cholinergic markers in neocortex lesioned with methylazoxymethanol acetate. J Neurochem 34:1429–1441.

14. Johnston MV, Grzanna R, Coyle JT (1979): Methylazoxymethanol treatment of fetal rats results in abnormally dense noradrenergic innervation of neocortex. Science 203:369–371.

15. Johnston MV, McKinney M, Coyle JT (1979): Evidence for a cholinergic projection to neocortex from neurons in the basal forebrain. Proc Natl Acad Sci USA 10:5392–5396.

16. Klein DF, Davis JM (eds) (1969): Diagnosis and Drug Treatment of Psychiatric Disorders. Baltimore, Williams & Wilkins.

17. Lauder J, Bloom FE (1974): Ontogeny of monoamine neurons in the locus coeruleus, raphe nuclei and substantia nigra of the rat. I. Cell differentiation. J Comp Neurol 155:469–482.

18. Moore RY, Bloom FE (1979): Central catecholamine neurosystems: anatomy and physiology of norepinephrine and epinephrine system. Ann Rev Neurosci 2:113–168.

19. Morrison JH, Grzanna R, Molliver ME, Coyle JT (1978): The distribution and orientation of noradrenergic fibers in the neocortex of the rat: An immunofluorescence study. J Comp Neurol 181:17–40.

20. Morrison JH, Molliver ME, Grzanna R (1979): Noradrenergic innervation of cerebral cortex: widespread effects of local cortical lesions. Science 205:313–316.

21. Ribac CE (1978): Aspinous and sparsely-spinous stellate neurons in the visual cortex of rats contain glutamic acid decarboxylase. Neurocytology 7:461–478.

22. Sastry BVR, Olubadervo J, Harbison RD, Schmidt DE (1976): Human placental cholinergic system. Occurrence, distribution and variation with gestational age of acetylcholine in human placenta. Biochem Pharmacol 25:425–431.

23. Schultz B, Nowak B, Maurer W (1974): Cycle times of neural epithelial cells of various types of neurons in the rat. An autoradiographic study. J Comp Neurol 158:207–218.

24. Shute C, Lewis PR (1967): The ascending cholinergic reticular system: neocortical, olfactory and subcortical projection. Brain 90:497–520.

25. Spatz M, Lacquer GL (1968): Transplacental chemical induction of microencephaly in two strains of rats. Proc Soc Exp Biol Med 129:705–710.

5

DEVELOPMENTAL NEUROPSYCHOPHARMACOLOGY: PRECLINICAL AND CLINICAL STUDIES OF THE HYPERKINETIC SYNDROME

George Breese, Thomas Gualtieri, Richard Mailman, Robert Mueller, William Youngblood, Richard Vogel, and Janet Wilson

The primary goals of psychiatric and neurologic research are to understand the etiology and neural mechanisms of disorders of the central nervous system (CNS) and to develop effective treatments for these diseases. Since technical and ethical constraints generally restrict human research related to central disorders, studies in animals to define the underlying bases of human disorders have become an important strategy. Our laboratory has been particularly interested in studies relevant to a developmental syndrome referred to as hyperkinesis (34), minimal brain dysfunction (MBD) (45), or attention deficit disorder (40). There is some doubt that a "complete" model of the hyperkinetic syndrome can be induced in animals (11). For this reason, two approaches have been undertaken in an effort to define the neural mechanisms involved in the hyperkinetic syndrome. The first strategy is to examine the mechanism(s) of action of amphetamine and methylphenidate, central stimulants effective in controlling symptoms of this disorder. The second approach is to define in animal models the involvement of neurotransmitter systems in specific functions, such as activity and impulse control, which are aberrant in children with MBD. The elucidation of the importance of monoamines in the action of d-amphetamine and the demonstration that hyperactivity can be induced in juvenile animals after neonatal interruption of mono-

From the Biological Sciences Research Center, University of North Carolina School of Medicine, Chapel Hill, North Carolina.
Supported by USPHS grants HD-10570 and HD-03110.

amine pathways will illustrate these approaches. In addition, a new animal model of impaired impulse control, a prominent symptom of the hyperkinetic syndrome, is described.

Our laboratory has recently complemented the basic mechanistic explorations in animals with studies in children designed to investigate the widely known variability in response to drug therapy of MBD. One aspect of this work was to test the hypothesis that the failure to obtain a therapeutic response to CNS stimulants in some hyperkinetic children may be caused by differences in drug disposition or metabolism rather than to different neurochemical bases of the disorder.

ROLE OF CATECHOLAMINE-CONTAINING SYSTEMS IN THE ACTIONS OF CENTRAL STIMULANTS

Since the central stimulants are useful therapeutically in the treatment of the hyperkinetic syndrome (1, 2), several studies have been undertaken to define the neural pathways involved in the locomotor stimulant actions of d-amphetamine and methylphenidate. Early work demonstrated that α-methyl-tyrosine, an inhibitor of tyrosine hydroxylase, antagonized the stimulant effects of d-amphetamine (24). Therefore, the initial efforts of

FIGURE 1. Effect of α-methyltyrosine (α-MPT) and U-14,624 on (A) d-amphetamine and (B) methylphenidate-induced motor activity in rats given reserpine. All rats received 2.5 mg/kg of reserpine 24 hours before receiving d-amphetamine sulfate (2 mg/kg) or methylphenidate (5 mg/kg). α-MPT (25 mg/kg) or U-14,624 (75 mg/kg) was administered at the beginning of the habituation (H) period, 1 hour before the stimulant drugs. (Modified from work by Hollister et al. [25] and Breese et al. [4].)

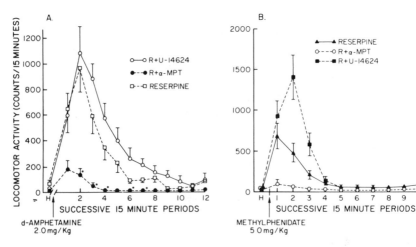

our laboratory focused on the involvement of catecholamine pathways in this action (6, 18, 19). Figure 1 shows that the locomotor stimulant action of both d-amphetamine and methylphenidate is reduced by α-methyltyrosine in rats treated with reserpine. In contrast, inhibition of norepinephrine synthesis with U-14,624 (an inhibitor of dopamine-β-hydroxylase) not only fails to block the action of the central stimulants but actually enhances the locomotor stimulant effects of methylphenidate (4, 25). This shows that dopaminergic, but not noradrenergic, pathways are critical for stimulant-induced increases in locomotor activity in rats. Further, the enhancement of the effects of methylphenidate after reduction of noradrenergic function demonstrates that released norepinephrine may have an inhibitory action in the control of locomotor activity.

Thus, indirect evidence exists that dopaminergic fibers are important for the locomotor stimulation induced by d-amphetamine. Therefore, more direct experiments were undertaken using 6-hydroxydopamine (with appropriate pharmacological manipulations) to destroy preferentially catecholamine-containing fibers within the CNS (3, 12, 13). As shown in Figure 2, the selective destruction of dopaminergic pathways results in a dramatic decrease in the locomotor stimulation induced by d-amphetamine (25), a finding consistent with the interpretation of our previous indirect pharmacologic manipulations (4, 25).

FIGURE 2. Effect of various 6-hydroxydopamine treatments on d-amphetamine-induced activity. Treatments are those described by Hollister et al. (25). *$p < .01$; **$p < .001$ when compared to control.

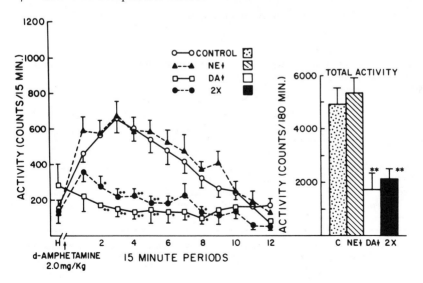

COMPARISONS OF CENTRAL STIMULANTS
WITH DOPAMINERGIC AGONISTS

Since the foregoing information suggests the stimulant action of d-amphetamine is related to endogenous dopamine release, it can be surmised that agents acting directly on dopaminergic receptors would mimic the effects of the central stimulants. Thus, such agents would be expected to act similarly to dopamine in biochemical tests of dopaminergic function. However, a series of investigations demonstrated these agonist drugs do not always have the predicted effect on either biochemical or physiologic measures of dopamine receptor activation (10, 28).

As shown in Table 1, the locomotor response to several agonist compounds in 6-hydroxydopamine-treated rats was found to be potentiated, consistent with the view that these drugs are acting on supersensitive dopaminergic receptors (23, 42). In agreement with earlier findings (25), the response to d-amphetamine was attenuated. However, the actions of these compounds to increase guanosine-3',5'-monophosphate (cGMP) in the cerebellum was varied. While d-amphetamine and apomorphine increased the content of cGMP in the cerebellum, the dopamine receptor agonists, lergotrile, piribedil, and bromocriptine, were without effect on this in vivo measure (10). Further, dopamine is known to stimulate adenylate cyclase activity in striatal homogenates. However, lergotrile, piribedil, and bromocriptine not only failed to stimulate the enzyme but actually inhibited the stimulant action of dopamine (Table 2). Finally, the agonist drugs differed markedly in their potency to displace H^3-spiperone bound to striatal tissue (Table 2) (28). As a compound with an indirect action, d-amphetamine was without effect on these measures.

Such data are consistent with the view that there are several types of dopamine receptors, as has been postulated previously by other investi-

TABLE 1. Effects of d-Amphetamine and Dopamine Agonists on Locomotor Activity and Cerebellar cGMP

Treatment	Dose (mg/kg)	Locomotor activity After 6-OHDA treatment (counts/150 min)	Cerebellar cGMP[a] (pmol/mg protein)
Saline	—	250 ± 45	8.8 ± 0.4
d-Amphetamine	1.0	425 ± 50	24.0 ± 2.5^b
Lergotrile	7.5	$13,437 \pm 4052^b$	8.5 ± 0.5
Piribedil	7.5	6788 ± 1916^b	6.4 ± 0.8
Bromocriptine	5.0	$19,375 \pm 2925^b$	8.8 ± 0.8
Apomorphine	3.0	6164 ± 940^b	24.0 ± 1.3^b

[a]Rats were killed 15 min after apomorphine and 30 min after the other drugs for measurement of cerebellar cGMP. Rats were allowed to habituate to the activity chamber for 1 hour before drug administration.

[b]$p < .01$ when compared to saline.

TABLE 2. Effects of Drugs Altering Dopaminergic Mechanisms on Dopamine Stimulated Adenylate Cyclase and ^{3}H-Spiperone Binding

Drug	Dopamine stimulated adenylate cyclase K_I (nM)[a]	^{3}H-spiperone displacement K_I (nM)[b]
d-Amphetamine	>21.2	>6000.0
Lergotrile	1.1	29.7
Piribedil	>21.2[c]	233.0
Bromocriptine	>21.2	0.5
Apomorphine	1.0	21.2

Values are determined from five duplications.

[a]K_I calculated from inhibition by the drug when the enzyme was stimulated with 50 μm dopamine.

[b]K_I calculated from experiments in which 0.65 nM ^{3}H-spiperone was used.

[c]K_I for piribedil has been determined to be 223 nM.

gators based on a variety of experimental approaches (17, 27, 41; see also Chapter 4). An intrinsic concern of our research is the possibility that only a specific subset of dopamine receptors is primarily responsible for the effects of d-amphetamine in the treatment of hyperkinesis. If this were the case, it might be possible to develop compounds that would more specifically produce the therapeutic effect of d-amphetamine while reducing the detrimental side effects described for the central stimulants in the treatment of the hyperkinetic syndrome (32, 33).

EXAMINATION OF THE ROLE OF SEROTONERGIC PATHWAYS IN THE ACTIONS OF CENTRAL STIMULANTS

An alternative explanation for the acknowledged clinical benefits obtained with the central stimulants is that they act on other neural systems as well as the catecholamine pathways. Therefore, in addition to studies in which our laboratory has examined the role of catecholamine-containing fibers in the action of central stimulants, other investigations examined the possibility that serotonin-containing fibers might influence the locomotor stimulant effects of this drug class (4, 5, 7, 26). For example, early work demonstrated that administration of pargyline (an MAO inhibitor) 1 hour before the injection of d-amphetamine or methylphenidate reduces the locomotor response to these stimulants (4, 5, 7). This antagonistic effect of pargyline is reversed by p-chlorophenylalanine (PCPA), an inhibitor of serotonin synthesis (4, 5). Thus, it appeared that serotonergic fibers exert an inhibitory influence on the activity induced by these stimulant drugs. Further support for this viewpoint was obtained when we found that reducing serotonin content with PCPA potentiates the locomotor stimulation induced by d-amphetamine and methylphenidate (Table 3) (4, 5).

TABLE 3. Effect of p-Chlorophenylalanine (PCPA) on d-Amphetamine and Methylphenidate Induced Locomotor Activity

Treatment	Locomotor activity (counts/180 min)
Saline	560 ± 50
d-Amphetamine	5670 ± 371
Methylphenidate	3660 ± 550
PCPA plus d-amphetamine	10,006 ± 1070[a]
PCPA plus methylphenidate	8440 ± 650[a]

Animals received a dose of 150 mg/kg of PCPA on two successive days before receiving d-amphetamine (3 mg/kg) or methylphenidate (10 mg/kg). The central stimulants were administered 24 hours after the last dose of PCPA. (Modified from Refs. [4, 26].)

[a] $p < .01$ when compared with d-amphetamine response.

Furthermore, a tryptophan-free diet, which decreases the function of serotonergic fibers by limiting the availability of the essential precursor, enhances the effects of d-amphetamine on locomotor activity (Figure 3) (26). This latter effect is reversed by pretreating the tryptophan deficient animals with tryptophan (Figure 4) (26). These data provide strong evidence that modulation of serotonergic function could alter the actions of d-amphetamine.

FIGURE 3. Effect of tryptophan-free diet on d-amphetamine-induced motor activity: time-course effect of the tryptophan-free diet on the locomotor response to 2.0 mg/kg d-amphetamine sulfate. Zero-day treatment represents the control response to d-amphetamine. Values represent the mean ± SEM of at least eight animals. Solid portion of the bars represents the activity accumulated for 3 hours to d-amphetamine. (From work by Hollister et al. [26].)

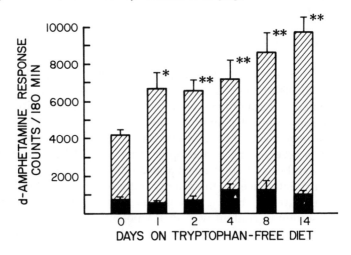

TABLE 4. Brain Content of Amphetamine in Rats Given a Tryptophan-Free Diet or PCPA Treatment

Treatment	Brain amphetamine (percent of control)
Saline	100 ± 5.2
PCPA (2 × 150 mg/kg)	106 ± 4.5
Tryptophan ↓ diet	93 ± 6.0

Content of d-amphetamine was measured 1 hour after injection of 2 mg/kg d-amphetamine sulfate. Levels of d-amphetamine in control animals was 10.3 ± 0.5. Each value represents the mean ± SEM of at least six animals. (Modified from Ref. [26].)

Since it is possible that the treatments altering serotonergic function might also alter the biotransformation of d-amphetamine, one additional experiment examined this possibility. The results presented in Table 4 indicate that neither p-chlorophenylalanine nor the tryptophan-free diet affects the content of d-amphetamine in brain. Thus, the enhancement of the action of d-amphetamine does not result from alterations in the metabolism or disposition of this central stimulant (26).

FIGURE 4. Reversal of tryptophan-free diet potentiation of d-amphetamine by L-tryptophan administration. Animals fed the tryptophan-free diet for 0, 1, 2, or 14 days received 100, 25, 25 and 100 mg/kg of L-tryptophan, respectively, 1 hour before administration of d-amphetamine. Values represent the mean ± SEM of at least eight rats. # $p < .05$; † $p < .01$ when compared with the no tryptophan treatment. (Data from Hollister et al. [26].)

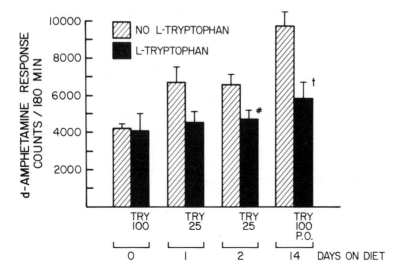

EFFECT OF MONOAMINE ALTERATIONS IN BRAIN
ON SPONTANEOUS LOCOMOTOR ACTIVITY

Investigations of the role of monoamine-containing pathways in the actions of the central stimulants demonstrate that dopaminergic, noradrenergic, and serotonergic pathways are all important in mediating the locomotor activity of these compounds. The question raised was whether alterations in monoamine function would result in hyperkinesis. One technique used to evaluate this possibility was to interrupt monoamine pathways in the neonate and examine the subsequent effect on locomotor activity (36).

As shown by earlier reports by Shaywitz and coworkers (36, 37), preferential reduction of brain dopamine with 6-hydroxydopamine causes a significant increase in locomotor activity during habituation (first 50 minutes) to the activity cages when the rats are 20 days of age (Table 5). However, at the time these rats are 40 to 60 days of age, activity is near or below control levels (21, 38). Preferential reduction of norepinephrine also results in hyperactivity at 20 days of age; however, this alteration is still apparent at 40 to 50 days of age (38). Similar experiments using 5,7-dihydroxytryptamine (5,7-DHT) demonstrated that a preferential reduction of serotonin in the neonate (8, 14, 15) causes locomotor activity to be elevated in rats at 14 but not 28 days of age (14).

Since central stimulants reduce hyperactivity in children (1, 44), the effects of d-amphetamine were examined against the hyperactivity observed in the various treatment groups. As shown in Table 5, the usual increase in locomotor activity caused by d-amphetamine is absent in those rats whose brain dopamine has been reduced, although Shaywitz et al.

TABLE 5. Effect of Interruption of Monoamines in the Neonate on Juvenile Activity

Treatment	Age tested	Locomotor activity (counts/50 min)	
		Saline	d-Amphetamine
Pargyline	14	218 ± 34^a	1118 ± 170^b
5-HT ↓	14	698 ± 77^a	1274 ± 80^b
DMI	20	608 ± 68	1241 ± 1120^b
DA ↓	20	1181 ± 152^a	1201 ± 144^b
NE ↓	20	1057 ± 130^a	2005 ± 203^b

For the group referred to as 5-HT ↓, rats received 50 µg of 5,7-dihydroxytryptamine (5,7-DHT) intracisternally (IC) 30 minutes after pargyline (40 mg/kg IP) at 3 days of age. The 6-OHDA (100 µg) was administered IC 60 minutes after DMI (20 mg/kg IP) at 3 days of age and this group is referred to as DA ↓. NE ↓ treatment group received 10 and 15 µg of 6-OHDA on days 1 and 3 after birth, respectively. Each value is the mean ± SEM of at least 12 determinations. (Data modified from Ref. [9, 14].)

$^a p < .05$ when compared to appropriate control group.

$^b p < .05$ when compared to activity in saline group.

(36) had shown previously that d-amphetamine in fact reduces the elevated activity in this group. Our results seem to agree with those of Eastgate et al. (20), who showed that 6-hydroxydopamine treatment reduces the elevation in activity induced by methylphenidate. In rats whose brain serotonin is reduced, d-amphetamine produces an increase in locomotor activity comparable to the effect in pargyline-treated control animals (Table 5). A greater than normal response in activity to d-amphetamine was noted in animals whose norepinephrine-containing fibers are destroyed. The latter response is consistent with earlier work suggesting that noradrenergic fibers may have an inhibitory function (4). However, the finding in rats depleted of brain serotonin neonatally does not agree with earlier findings that depletion of brain serotonin in adult rats enhances the locomotor stimulation induced by d-amphetamine (4).

Recent clinical data demonstrated that both normal boys and those with hyperkinetic syndrome show reduced locomotion after d-amphetamine (30). In our experimental paradigm, there was no indication that d-amphetamine reduces locomotor activity in normal neonatal rats. Most investigators have suggested that an animal model of the hyperkinetic syndrome should demonstrate a reduction of locomotor activity following the administration of stimulant drugs. Perhaps the clinical data challenge this concept. For example, it is possible that rats and humans have a qualitatively different response to low doses of stimulants. This consideration makes it difficult to judge whether stimulant-induced reduction in activity in the animal models of hyperactivity should even be expected. Regardless, these animal models indicate how interruption of several neural systems can lead to hyperactivity and, at the very least, probably have relevance to those children who do not respond favorably to the stimulant drugs.

EVALUATION OF MODELS OF IMPULSE CONTROL

Most efforts to develop animal models of the hyperkinetic syndrome have focused on reproducing the hyperactivity of the syndrome, while ignoring other prominent clinical symptoms such as distractibility, short attention span, excitability, and impulsivity, even though these latter symptoms may be more central to the disorder than the hyperactivity. For this reason, we have begun recently to examine neural mechanisms pertinent to impulse control in two different behavioral paradigms involving the ability of rats to suppress responses that lead to mild punishment. This approach was taken with the view that these behaviors may be homologous to the characteristics of impulse control in humans.

The first model of impulse control, a passive avoidance procedure, has been used to evaluate the effect of preferential reduction of brain catecholamines on the animal's ability to inhibit responding (Table 6). In this

TABLE 6. Effect of 6-Hydroxydopamine Treatments on Passive Avoidance Responding

Treatment	Latency to enter shock compartment[a]		
	Training trial	Retest trial after shock	Retest trial after no shock
Saline	11.4 ± 3.0	177 ± 3.4	10.2 ± 1.6
6-OHDA	9.2 ± 1.0	170 ± 10.1	15.8 ± 2.0
DA ↓	8.9 ± 1.6	148 ± 13.2	7.5 ± 1.3
NE ↓	8.5 ± 2.1	113 ± 20.1[b]	5.8 ± 2.0

[a]Values represent the mean latency ± SEM in seconds to enter the shock compartment. There are at least 12 rats in each group. The 6-OHDA group received 100 μg 6-hydroxydopamine (6-OHDA) at 5 days of age. The DA ↓ group received 20 mg/kg of desipramine 1 hour before receiving 100 μg of 6-OHDA. The NE ↓ group received 15 μg and 25 μg of 5-OHDA on 3 and 5 days, respectively. (Unpublished data and Ref. [6].)

[b]$p < .05$ when compared to saline group.

regard, reduction of norepinephrine in the neonate causes a significant deficit in this task when the rats are approximately 50 days old, whereas dopamine depletion is without effect. However, the alteration noted after destruction of noradrenergic pathways does not appear to be a learning deficiency per se, because similar modification of noradrenergic function does not impair acquisition in an active avoidance paradigm (38). Thus, this evaluation of impulse control would implicate noradrenergic systems in this symptom of the hyperkinetic syndrome. It would also be interesting to analyze the effect of disrupting serotonergic fibers on this measure, but these studies have not yet been conducted.

The other approach to developing a model of deficient impulse control is the use of pharmacologic agents that reduce the capacity of an animal to inhibit behavioral responding when punished (43). In these conflict (approach–avoidance) paradigms, chlordiazepoxide has been shown to disinhibit the suppression of responding caused by punishment (35, 43). Thus, it is possible to describe the action of the benzodiazepines in a conflict task as a functional deficit of attenuated impulse control—a situation analogous to the impulsivity observed in MBD. In this regard, benzodiazepines have been reported to have unfavorable action in the hyperkinetic syndrome (46). Nonetheless, if this paradigm is to be a useful model of impulse control, drugs that are beneficial in the treatment of the hyperkinetic syndrome should reverse the deficit induced by the benzo-diazepines and drugs like phenobarbital should worsen it. As shown in Table 7, d-amphetamine reduced the deficit induced by chlordiazepoxide in the conflict paradigm, whereas phenobarbital worsened the ability of the rat to inhibit responding. Thus, this experimental model of impulse control may be useful for preclinical testing of the potential efficacy of drugs in the hyperkinetic syndrome. In addition, the work further suggests

TABLE 7. Effects of d-Amphetamine and Phenobarbital on the Chlordiazepoxide Induced Increase in Responding in a Conflict Paradigm

Treatment	Dose (mg/kg)	Responses (shocks/3 min)
Saline	—	6.0 ± 1.0
Chlordiazepoxide (CDZ)	8.0	15.1 ± 3.1^a
CDZ plus d-amphetamine	8 + 1.0	8.9 ± 2.7^b
d-Amphetamine	1.0	6.3 ± 1.5
CDZ plus phenobarbital	8 + 5.0	$26.0 \pm 2.0^{a,b}$
Phenobarbital	5.0	18.3 ± 8.8^a

Rats were injected intraperitoneally with saline or the other drugs 30 minutes before testing. The procedure used is a modification of that described by Vogel et al. (43). There are at least 12 rats in each group

$^a p < 0.05$ when compared to saline.

$^b p < 0.05$ when compared to CDZ treatment only.

that efforts to influence neural systems critical to the actions of the benzodiazepines may provide important insights into the neurobiology of impulse control.

EVALUATION OF METHYLPHENIDATE IN SERUM OF MBD CHILDREN

Even though the therapeutic effect of central stimulants among children with the hyperkinetic syndrome was central to the recognition of this central disorder (2), only a few investigators have studied carefully the different aspects of the clinical response to the central stimulants. For example, Sprague et al. (39) observed a dissociation between the cognitive and behavioral effects of different doses of methylphenidate among hyperactive children. Recently, Rapoport and coworkers (30) found that normal boys showed the same behavioral responses to d-amphetamine as hyperactive boys. These latter clinical studies have been extremely important, since they are indicative of how knowledge of drug response can enhance our understanding of the biology of childhood hyperkinesis.

In spite of the documented effectiveness of the central stimulants in the treatment of the hyperkinetic syndrome (1, 39), not all hyperkinetic children gain therapeutic advantage when treated with the central stimulants. It is known that lack of responsiveness to other psychotropic drugs can be related to differences in drug metabolism. Therefore, our laboratory has sought to determine if the lack of methylphenidate effectiveness among some hyperkinetic children could be attributed to an altered pharmacokinetic pattern in these patients. This is an extremely important question, because if the difference cannot be attributed to changes in drug metabolism, it would suggest a lack of homogeniety within the group of children diagnosed as having the hyperkinetic syndrome. A sensitive assay for methylphenidate levels in blood, using gas chromatographic separation and quantitative measurement with a mass spectrometer, has been developed for investigating this problem.

Following oral administration (0.3 mg/kg methylphenidate), the level of this drug found in plasma of ten adult normal individuals at various times over a 6 hour period is shown in Figure 5. Peak levels of methylphenidate occurred in these subjects within 60 to 90 minutes after administration, with substantial levels still present at 6 hours. Within this limited population, the maximal content in serum varied from 3 to 24 ng/ml. This wide range of interindividual variation in maximal methylphenidate concentration has been confirmed in other studies conducted in 41 individuals (19 hyperactive children and 22 normal adults). Values in these subjects ranged from 1.1 to 21.6 ng/ml of serum 1 hour after oral administration of 0.3 mg/kg of methylphenidate.

We have also attempted to relate serum levels of methylphenidate to the therapeutic response of 15 hyperkinetic children using a double-blind, cross-over design. Only one dose of methylphenidate (0.3 mg/kg) was used in this experiment and serum levels were measured 1 hour after oral administration. Clinical response was rated using the Conner's rating scale, as well as a global consensus based on impressions of parents, physicians, and teachers. In addition to these subjective measures, objective measures of drug response were also made. The continuous performance task was

FIGURE 5. Serum levels of methlyphenidate after oral administration to ten adult males.

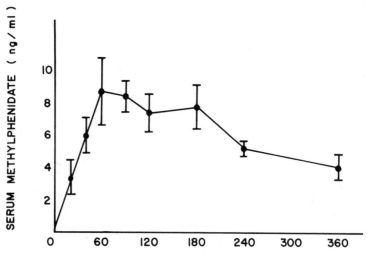

TIME AFTER ADMINISTRATION
OF 0.3mg/kg METHYLPHENIDATE
(min)

TABLE 8. Hyperkinetic Syndrome: Serum Content and Laboratory Measures after Methylphenidate Administration[a]

| Classification | n | Serum methyl- phenidate (ng/ml) | Global behavior | Continuous performance responses[b] | | Growth hormone[b] (ng/ml) |
				correct	incorrect	
Responder	6	6.8 ± 1.6	Improved	21.5 ± 4.5	24.3 ± 7.2	5.8 ± 3.2
Nonresponder	9	9.9 ± 2.4	Not improved	8.4 ± 5.4	22.0 ± 11.0	4.5 ± 1.5

[a]Measures of growth hormone and serum methylphenidate were made 60 minutes after oral administration of methylphenidate (0.3 mg/kg). The continuous performance testing occurred 60 to 90 minutes after treatment. Global behavior assessment was made 1 week after initiation of the methylphenidate therapy.

[b]Values are changed from measure obtained when individual received saline.

used to measure attention (vigilance) (29), and the movement in a laboratory playroom provided a measure of gross motor activity in a free field playroom situation (31). The incremental change in growth hormone levels provided a physiologic measure of the action of methylphenidate (16). The results of this study are presented in Table 8. Whereas six children responded to methylphenidate (responders), the behavior in nine children did not improve (nonresponders). However, the group of hyperkinetic children who responded to methylphenidate had serum levels of methylphenidate comparable to those children whose behavior did not improve. Further, the drug was apparently exerting a central effect among the nine children who were not good clinical responders because objective measures showed changes that were similar to those seen among the responders. The conclusions that can be drawn from these data must be considered to be tentative, since a larger group of children must be studied at different doses before any definitive statements can be made. Nevertheless, the results are consistent with the view that there is biologic heterogeneity among hyperactive children (22).

SUMMARY

This overview illustrated how a multidisciplinary program, using both clinical and preclinical expertise, can increase our understanding of a central disorder. We examined both the mechanism of action of central stimulants and the symptoms of the disease in animal models to generate hypotheses concerning the role of neurotransmitter systems in the hyperkinetic syndrome. For example, the monoamine systems were found to contribute to the stimulant action of d-amphetamine, and interruption of each of the monoamine systems in the neonate led to increased locomotor activity. Such data suggest the possible involvement of dopaminergic, noradrenergic, and serotonergic systems in the symptoms of the hyperkinetic syndrome. Other experiments sought to evaluate the symptoms of impulsivity demonstrated in MBD. Impulse control was determined in paradigms that examine the ability of rats to suppress responding that leads to mild punishment. Finally, evaluation of the pharmacokinetics of methylphenidate in children with MBD shows that serum levels in children who respond therapeutically to this drug are similar to those that do not.

Collectively, the preclinical and clinical findings support the hypothesis that the symptoms of the hyperkinetic syndrome may not have a single pathophysiologic basis. Future work will continue to examine this perspective, because this knowledge may facilitate development of treatments for children who do not respond to stimulant drugs. Furthermore, by increasing the homogeneity of subgroups within the hyperkinetic syndrome, the chances of identifying abnormal molecular processes should be enhanced.

REFERENCES AND BIBLIOGRAPHY

1. Barkley RA (1977): A review of stimulant drug research with hyperactive children. J Child Psychol 18:137–165.
2. Bradley C (1937): Behavior of children receiving benzedrine. Am J Psychiatry 94: 577–585.
3. Breese GR, Cooper BR (1977): Chemical lesioning: Catecholamine pathways. Meth Psychobiol 3:27–46.
4. Breese GR, Cooper BR, Hollister AS (1975): Involvement of brain monoamines in the stimulant and paradoxical inhibitory effects of methylphenidate. Psychopharmacologia 44:5–10.
5. Breese GR, Cooper BR, Mueller RA (1974): Evidence for involvement of 5-hydroxytryptamine in the actions of amphetamine. Br J Pharmacol 52:307–314.
6. Breese GR, Cooper BR, Smith RD (1973): Biochemical and behavioral alterations following 6-hydroxydopamine administration into brain. In Usden E, Snyder S, eds: Frontiers in Catecholamine Research. New York, Pergamon Press, pp 701–706.
7. Breese GR, Hollister AS, Cooper BR (1976): Role of monoamine neural pathways in d-amphetamine- and methylphenidate-induced locomotor activity. In Ellenwood EH Jr, Kilbey MM, eds: Cocaine and Other Stimulants. New York, Plenum, pp 445–455.
8. Breese GR, Mueller RA (1978): Alterations in the neurocytotoxicity of 5,7-dihydroxytryptamine by pharmacological agents in adult and developing rats. Ann NY Acad Sci 305:160–174.
9. Breese GR, Mueller RA, Lipton MA (1978): Developmental neuropsychopharmacology. In Lipton M, DiMascio A, Killam K, eds: Psychopharmacology—A Generation of Progress. New York, Raven Press, pp 609–620.
10. Breese GR, Mueller RA, Mailman RB (1979): Effect of dopaminergic agonists and antagonists on in vivo cyclic nucleotide content: Relation of cerebellar cGMP changes to behavior. J Pharmacol Exp Ther 209:262–270.
11. Breese GR, Mueller RA, Mailman RB, Frye GD, Vogel RA (1978): Study of drug mechanisms and disease symptoms: Alternatives to animal models of CNS disorders. Prog Neuropsychopharmacol 2:313–325.

12. Breese GR, Traylor TD (1971): Depletion of brain noradrenaline and dopamine by 6-hydroxydopamine. Br J Pharmacol 42:88–99.

13. Breese GR, Traylor TD (1970): Effect of 6-hydroxydopamine on brain norepinephrine and dopamine: Evidence for selective degeneration of catecholamine neurons. J Pharmacol Exp Ther 174:413–420.

14. Breese GR, Vogel RA, Mueller RA (1978): Biochemical and behavioral alterations in developing rats treated with 5,7-dihydroxytryptamine. J Pharmacol Exp Ther 205:587–595.

15. Breese GR, Vogel RA, Kuhn CM, Mailman RB, Mueller RA, Schanberg SM (1978): Behavioral and prolactin responses to 5-hydroxytryptophan in rats treated during development with 5,7-dihydroxytryptamine. Brain Res 155:263–275.

16. Brown WA (1977): Psychologic and neuroendocrine response to methylphenidate. Arch Gen Psychiatry 34:1103–1108.

17. Cools AR, Van Rossum JM (1976): Excitation-mediating and inhibition-mediating dopamine receptors: A new concept towards a better understanding of electrophysiological, biochemical, pharmacological, functional and clinical data. Psychopharmacologia 45:243–254.

18. Cooper BR, Cott JM, Breese GR (1974): Effects of catecholamine-depleting drugs and amphetamine on self-stimulation of brain following various 6-hydroxydopamine treatments. Psychopharmacologia 37:235–248.

19. Cooper BR, Konkol RJ, Breese GR (1978): Effects of catecholamine depleting drugs and d-amphetamine on self-stimulation of the substantia nigra and locus coeruleus. J Pharmacol Exp Ther 204:592–605.

20. Eastgate SM, Wright JJ, Werry JS (1978): Behavioural effects of methylphenidate in 6-hydroxydopamine-treated neonatal rats. Psychopharmacology 58:157–159.

21. Erinoff L, Macphail RC, Heller A, Seiden LS (1979): Age-dependent effects of 6-hydroxydopamine on locomotor activity in the rat. Brain Res 164:195–205.

22. Fish B (1971): The "one child, one drug" myth of stimulants in hyperkinesis. Arch Gen Psychiatry 25:193–203.

23. Fuxe K, Fredholm BB, Ögren S-O, Agnati LF, Hökfelt T, Gustafsson J-Å (1978): Ergot drug and central monoaminergic mechanisms: A histochemical, biochemical and behavioral analysis. Fed Proc 37:2181–2191.

24. Hanson LCF (1966): Evidence that the central action of amphetamine is mediated via catecholamines. Psychopharmacologia 9:78–80.

25. Hollister AS, Breese GR, Cooper BR (1974): Comparison of tyrosine hydroxylase and dopamine-β-hydroxylase inhibition with the effects of various 6-hydroxydopamine treatments on d-amphetamine induced motor activity. Psychopharmacologia 36:1–16.

26. Hollister AS, Breese GR, Kuhn CM, Cooper BR, Schanberg SM (1976): An inhibitory role for brain serotonin-containing systems in the locomotor effects of d-amphetamine. J Pharmacol Exp Ther 198:12–22.

27. Kebabian JW, Calne DB (1979): Multiple receptors for dopamine. Nature 277:93–96.

28. Kilts CD, Smith DA, Ondrusek MG, Mailman RB, Mueller RA, Breese GR (1979): Differential effects of "dopaminergic agonists" on measures of dopaminergic function. Neurosci Abst 5:647.

29. Mirsky AF, Gordon PV (1962): A comparison of the behavioural and physiological changes accompanying sleep deprivation and chlorpromazine administration in man. Electroencephalogr Clin Neurophysiol 14:1–10.

30. Rapoport JL, Bachsbaum MS, Zahn TP, Weingartner H, Ludlow C, Mikkelsen EJ (1978): Dextroamphetamine: Cognitive and behavioral effects in normal prepubertal boys. Science 199:560–563.

31. Routh DK, Schroeder CS, O'Tuama L (1974): Development of activity level in children. Dev Psychol 10:163–168.

32. Safer D, Allen R, Barr E (1972): Depression of growth in hyperactive children on stimulant drugs. N Engl J Med 287:217–220.

33. Satterfield JH, Cantwell DP, Schell A, Blaschke T (1979): Growth of hyperactive children treated with methylphenidate. Arch Gen Psychiatry 36:212–217.

34. Schuckit MA, Petrich J, Chiles J (1978): Hyperactivity: Diagnostic confusion. J Nerv Ment Dis 166:79–87.

35. Sepinwall J, Cook L (1978): Behavioral pharmacology of anti-anxiety drugs. In Iversen LL, Iversen SD, Snyder SH, eds: Handbook of Psychopharmacology, vol. 13. New York, Plenum Press, pp 345–393.

36. Shaywitz BA, Klopper JH, Yager RD, Gordon JW (1976): Paradoxical response to amphetamine in developing rats treated with 6-hydroxydopamine. Nature 261:153–155.

37. Shaywitz BA, Yager RD, Klopper JH (1976): Selective brain dopamine depletion in developing rats: An experimental model of minimal brain dysfunction. Science 191:305–308.

38. Smith RD, Cooper BR, Breese GR (1973): Growth and behavioral changes in developing rats treated intracisternally with 6-hydroxydopamine: Evidence for involvement of brain dopamine. J Pharmacol Exp Ther 185:609–619.

39. Sprague RL, Sleator EK (1977): Methylphenidate in hyperkinetic children: Differences in dose effects on learning and social behavior. Science 198:1274–1276.

40. Task force on Nomenclature and Statistics of the American Psychiatric Association. DSM-III draft. American Psychiatric Association, Washington, DC, 15 January 1978.

41. Titeler M, Weinreich P, Sinclair D, Seeman P (1978): Multiple receptors for brain dopamine. Proc Natl Acad Sci USA 75:1153–1156.

42. Ungerstedt U (1971): Post synaptic supersensitivity after 6-hydroxydopamine induced degeneration of the nigrostriatal dopamine system. Acta Physiol Scand 367:79–93.

43. Vogel JR, Beer B, Clody DE (1971): A simple and reliable conflict procedure for testing anti-anxiety agents. Psychopharmacologia 21:1–7.

44. Wender PH (1975): The minimal brain dysfunction syndrome. Ann Rev Med 26:45–62.

45. Wender PH (1972): The minimal brain dysfunction syndrome in children. J Nerv Ment Dis 155:55–71.

46. Werry JS (1976): Medications for hyperkinetic children. Drugs 11:81–89.

6

MONOAMINE OXIDASE AND AGING

T. Peter Bridge, Steven Potkin, C. David Wise, Bruce H. Phelps, and Richard Jed Wyatt

Correlations, though never demonstrating causality, serve to stimulate scientific curiosity and investigation. One such correlation has been the observation of increased monoamine oxidase (MAO) activity with advancing age. Monoamine oxidase, an enzyme critical to the degradation of catechol compounds and many other biogenic amines, is found in multiple tissues and species. In addition to increases with advancing age, alterations of MAO activity have been demonstrated in several disease states. However, like advancing age, causal links between altered enzyme activity and disease state have not been demonstrated. The increase in MAO activity with advancing age is unlike most enzymes, which decrease in activity during senescence. This chapter is an effort to examine a number of areas of basic and clinical work that bear on the issue of altered monoaminergic function and the processes of aging.

HUMAN STUDIES OF MONOAMINE OXIDASE AND AGE

Although a specific assay for MAO has been available for nearly 20 years, it is only within the last decade that it has been widely used in demographically diverse populations and in a variety of clinical states (5). Such work has demonstrated that MAO has two apparent types, MAO-A and MAO-B that respond differentially to specific substrates and specific inhibitors (33). The seminal work with respect to platelet MAO and aging

Laboratory of Clinical Psychopharmacology, Division of Special Mental Health Research, Intramual Research Program, National Institute of Mental Health, Saint Elizabeths Hospital, Washington, D.C.

A. Raskin, D. S. Robinson, and J. Levine, eds., Age and the Pharmacology of Psychoactive Drugs.

was done by Robinson and colleagues (37, 45–47). They observed, from cross-sectional data, that males and females had increases in both plasma and platelet MAO activity after age 50. They also examined platelet and plasma MAO among a group of depressed individuals relative to controls and found that enzyme activity is elevated for both tissues (benzylamine was used as a substrate). In samples of hindbrain obtained at autopsy from a group of individuals who died from diverse causes (using both benzylamine and tryptamine as substrates), these workers found that the concentration of MAO activity was greater in all eight brain areas assayed, particularly the hypothalamus, for the older group (age > 45 years) relative to the younger subjects (age < 45 years). Curious about the possible relationship of brain MAO activity and brain monoamines, they measured 5-hydroxytryptamine (5-HT), 5-hydroxyindolacetic acid (5-HIAA), and norepinephrine (NE) in various brain regions. No alterations in either 5-HT or 5-HIAA content in hindbrain relative to age were observed. On the other hand, NE was decreased in hindbrain, an observation consistent with the observed increase of hindbrain MAO activity. In contrast, plasma NE has been observed to increase with advancing age. Ziegler et al. (54) also reported that older individuals have greater increases in plasma NE in response to stressful experiences.

After the work of Robinson et al. (46, 47), other investigators also examined cross-sectional data for age-related changes in MAO activity. These results have not been entirely consistent. Murphy et al. (33) did not observe correlations between platelet MAO activity and age (using benzylamine as a substrate) up to age 60 years. More recent work by Bridge et al. (7) with an assay using platelet pellets rather than platelet-rich plasma and tyramine as a substrate, demonstrated clear increases in activity with advancing age. (see Table 1). In examining patient data, Gershon et al. (20) did not see an age effect on plasma MAO activity in a group of patients with primary depressive disorder. Takahashi (50) also examined platelet MAO activity in both manic and depressed patients and failed to find any relationship between diagnostic group and enzyme activity relative to controls. Further, Takahashi did not observe any age effects on platelet MAO activity within the control group, nor did the group of depressed individuals have higher MAO activity relative to the

TABLE 1. Platelet Monoamine Oxidase Activity, by Age Group in a General Population

Age range (years)	n	Mean age	SEM	Platelet MAO	SEM	T
18–50	84	26.0	1.8	18.14	0.72	
51–79	32	61.9	1.9	25.45	1.35	5.15
						$p < .001$

manic group. He did not, however, report whether there was an age effect on platelet MAO activity in the depressed group. Murphy and Weiss (35) also failed to find any differences in platelet MAO activity for unipolar depressed patients but did, in contrast to Takahashi's work, find lowered platelet MAO activity in bipolar affective patients.

Among schizophrenic patients, many of whom show alterations of MAO activity relative to controls, Brockington et al. (8) failed to find any age effects upon platelet MAO activity for either schizophrenic or schizoaffective patients. Orsulak et al. (41) have noted that schizoaffective patients have higher platelet MAO activity relative to both controls and schizophrenic patients. They did not find evidence of age effects on enzyme activity in their sample. Bridge et al. (6), in contrast, studied a group of patients, aged 50 years and older, who had a research diagnostic criteria (RDC) diagnosis of chronic schizophrenia at admission and observed that those patients who demonstrated substantial symptomatic improvement had higher platelet MAO activity than those who failed to show significant improvement (see Table 2). Furthermore, within both the control and patient groups there was evidence of increasing platelet MAO activity with advancing age. Von Knooring et al. (51) studied platelet MAO activity and visual average evoked responses in a diverse group of psychiatrically ill patients and reported that both MAO types (A and B) increase in activity with advancing age for all patients. They also examined the relationship of age, enzyme activity, and the results of numerous neurophysiologic measures, but the diversity of diagnoses within the patient group makes it difficult to interpret their findings. In very young schizophrenics, however, no differences between patients and controls emerge for platelet MAO activity (11). Patients aged 10 years and under do show higher MAO activity than those aged 11 to 14 years and pubertal male patients have higher enzyme activity relative to controls.

TABLE 2. Platelet Monoamine Oxidase Activity in a Group of Patients Diagnosed at Admission as Schizophrenic by Research Diagnostic Criteria (RDC)

	Group 1: Normal controls	Group 2: Patients who presently do not merit RDC diagnosis of schizophrenia	Group 3: Patients who presently merit RDC diagnosis of schizophrenia
n	18	12	14
Mean age	69.5	72.7	71.9
SEM (age)	1.2	2.6	2.5
Platelet MAO nM/mg/hr	29.35	31.01	19.35
SEM (MAO)	2.01	1.38	1.4
P value	—	.51	.001

Evidence for age effects on MAO activity is also present in a study by Aldinio et al. (2) who examined controls and patients with glaucoma for platelet MAO activity. Although a difference in enzyme activity was found in the patient group compared to the controls, both groups had increases in enzyme activity in the older subjects. Female patients had higher activity than the males, and elevations of enzyme activity were seen for female subjects older then 40 and for male subjects older than 50.

Postmortem studies afford data concerning MAO activity within the central nervous system, although such studies are not without methodologic difficulties. Carlsson and Winblad (9) noted dopamine decreases in the basal ganglia with both advancing age and increasing time interval between moment of death and autopsy. Examination of postmortem material demonstrated decreased dopamine and NE in the hypothalamus, nucleus accumbens, putamen, and frontal cortex of the brains of the patients with senile dementia compared to the controls (1). Patients with senile dementia of the Alzheimer type have also been reported to have elevated platelet MAO activity relative to age matched controls (52). Autopsy material has also demonstrated elevated MAO activity in the brains of patients with senile dementia (Alzheimer type) relative to age-matched controls (52). Winblad et al. (53) examined platelet MAO activity antemortem in a group of nonpsychiatric nonneurologic geriatric patients and compared these findings with MAO activity of their postmortem brain tissue. Tissue from the hypothalamus, hippocampus, caudate, and cingulategyrus failed to show any relationship of brain MAO and platelet MAO activity. Because they used subjects without sufficient variance in age, they were unable to examine age effects. Owen et al. (42) did look at MAO activity in the brains of psychiatrically normal individuals and found enzyme activity to be highest in the nucleus accumbens. They were unable, however, to find age-related differences in types A and B MAO.

ANIMAL STUDIES OF MONOAMINE INHIBITORS AND AGE

Demonstration of alterations of MAO enzyme activity with advancing age in animal studies antedates the observation in humans. Novick (38) reported in 1961, that MAO activity is elevated in liver tissue of older rats compared to younger animals. Gey et al. (21) repeated this finding in 1965 and also reported that NE was decreased in the cardiac tissue of older rats. Prange and his colleagues (43) in 1967 found MAO activity elevated in both cardiac and brain tissue of older rats.

Horita (23) and Horita and Lowe (24) replicated the findings of increased MAO activity in cardiac tissue of older rats. This promising initial series of studies led investigators to look at other questions relating age and the monoaminergic systems. Gripois (22) reported on developmental issues with respect to MAO activity in the fetal rat. This investigator suggested that fetal MAO may be produced maternally, as intraamniotic injections of MAO inhibitors result in fetal death. At birth, however, the activity of MAO is approximately equal to adult levels for brain, kidney, liver, duodenum, and heart. In mice, however, only MAO type A is present at approximately adult levels at birth; MAO type B continues to increase from birth to day 24 postpartum before leveling off at adult levels (15). Radha (44) reported that among young rats there appears to be a circadian variation in MAO activity of brain tissue, depending on the time of day the animal is killed. He noted that MAO activity is highest at 8 am and that this pattern persists with advancing age of the animal. In contrast, the circadian peak of MAO inhibition of rat brain tissue by procaine HCl (Gerovital) increases with advancing age and shifts with increasing age from 12 pm to 4 pm.

In the last decade, the number of investigations of alterations of MAO activity and monoamines in other species and other tissues has expanded. To facilitate comparison of results from these studies, the findings are presented in Table 3. As can be seen, the results of these studies do not demonstrate consistency of age effects on MAO activity or monoamines.

In general, rat myocardium shows increases of MAO activity in older animals, although no such change is observed for either mice or rabbits (16, 17, 27, 44, 48). The results from rat liver tissue are variable, although the assays used are not comparable (19, 44, 48). Vascular tissues, except for cerebrovascular tissue, appear to have decreased MAO activity across the life span (17, 27). Cerebral vasculature both demonstrates the highest MAO activity of all vascular tissue and shows further increases in activity in older animals (27). Rat brain MAO activity increased in older animals, and apparently MAO type A has a greater increase in activity than MAO type B (44, 48, 49). Mice and rabbits do not, however, have cerebral changes in MAO activity nor in NE content (16). Rat brain, in contrast, has both increased MAO activity and decreased dopamine and NE content (49). Decreased NE sensitivity is also found in rat myocardium, which may represent a compensatory change for alterations observed in plasma NE (54). In rhesus monkeys, platelet MAO activity has been observed to be elevated among older male monkeys, but no such changes were seen in the older female monkeys (34).

For both animal and human studies, then, the data pertaining to the monoaminergic systems and older age groups are by no means consistent. Most of the evidence does suggest, however, that cardiac and brain tissues for rats have inceased MAO activity in older animals. Further, human data suggest that activity of MAO in platelet and brain tissue increases across the life span. With the human data in particular, the caveat must be borne in mind that these studies all represent cross-sectional data. No longitudinal observations have been made that demonstrate increasing MAO activity across the life span.

TABLE 3. MAO Activity in Aging Animals

Study	Year	Tissue (species)	MAO activity change with age	Amine content change with age
Radna (1978)	1978	Liver (rat)	↑	—
		Heart (rat)	↓	—
Feldman and Roche (1978)	1978	Liver Pancreas } Mice, Kidney } rabbit Brain	No change in MAO	— — —
Shih (1975)	1975	Liver (rat)	No change in MAO A and B (age 2–24 months)	—
		Brain (rat)	↑ MAO A and ↓ MAO B (age 2–4 months)	—
Gandhi and Kanungo (1974)	1974	Liver (rat)	↓	—
Fuentes et al. (1977)	1977	Heart (rat)	↑ A and B (↑ > A)	—
		Mesenteric artery (rat)	↓ A and B (A decr > B)	—
		Aorta	↓ A and B (A decr > B)	—
Lai et al. (1978)	1978	Heart (rat) Cerebral microvessels	↑ ↑, highest MAO for all tissues compared	— —
		Mesenteric artery	↑ to 3 weeks of age, then no change	—
Simpkins, Mueller, Huang and Meites (1977)	1977	Hypothalamus (rat)	—	Decrease dopamine; decrease norepine- phrine; 5 HT, no change
Murphy, Redmond, Beuller, Donnelly, Ziegler, Lake and Kopin (1978)	1976	Platelet (rhesus monkey)	↑ for males only	

GEROVITAL STUDIES

Another line of evidence, though more controversial than the data from enzyme studies, centers on the clinical use of buffered procaine HCL (Gerovital). European open trials claim this drug reverses age effects (3, 4). Hypertensive, arthritic, and depressive symptoms are said to be ameliorated by Gerovital. Gerovital has also been reported to prolong cellular proliferation of monkey and chick embryo cultures (40). Mouse fibroblast cultures treated with Gerovital during the proliferative phase had prolonged capacity to divide and proliferate compared to controls (39). Further, those cultures that had ceased to proliferate, when treated with Gerovital, could be maintained longer than controls. This evident reversal of the Hayflick effect (age-dependent limitation of fibroblast cell culture regeneration) is potentially attributed to the MAO inhibiting properties of Gerovital.

Gerovital is a reversible MAO inhibitor. It is reportedly more effective than commercial procaine as an MAO inhibitor in rat brain, but much less effective than iproniazid (31, 32). Procaine may also be a better type A than type B MAO inhibitor (18).

Clinical trials in the United States of Gerovital as an antidepressant produced mixed but generally negative results. Although Cohen and Ditman (10) reported that patients experienced relief of depressive symptoms in an open trial; double blind studies later failed to demonstrate any efficacy of Gerovital as an antidepressant, though in general, both treated and untreated patients improved (40, 55). The observation of Fuller and Rouse (18) that the reversibility of procaine's MAO inhibition makes it a less effective inhibitor may offer some explanation as to the failure to demonstrate any antidepressant effects of Gerovital.

MONOAMINERGIC PRECURSORS

Parkinson's disease has been demonstrated to be related to an alteration in the monoaminergic system. Anatomic alterations in the substantia nigra result in depletion of dopamine and cause parkinsonism. This has led to the treatment of parkinsonism with a precursor of dopamine (L-dopa) with generally good, though variable, clinical results. Since parkinsonism is usually a disease of the elderly, this treatment affords the opportunity to observe other interactions of the monoaminergic system and advanced age. One of the more intriguing observations has been that use of L-dopa, metabolized by MAO, is associated with increased longevity of Parkinson's disease patients (14). This may be caused by an observed decrease of intercurrent illnesses that were often fatal for patients with Parkinson's disease, since L-dopa does not appear to alter the course of Parkinson's disease otherwise. Further, L-dopa does not evidently affect the onset or development of dementia, which also characterizes parkinsonism (14). In contrast to the findings for other aged individuals, hypothalamic MAO activity has been found to be decreased in Parkinson's disease patients (36). These same investigators also reported decrease of other hypothalamic catecholamine related enzymes (dopamine beta hydroxylase (DBH) and phenylethanol N methyltransferase [PMNT]) in patients with Parkinson's disease relative to controls. It is interesting, however, that deprenyl, a specific MAO type B inhibitor, reduces the dosage of L-dopa required to achieve beneficial effect and also prolongs the effectiveness of L-dopa, presumably by reducing the rate of destruction of dopamine provided by L-dopa (28).

Although it is not efficacious in the treatment of Parkinson dementia, L-dopa has been administered to patients with senile dementia. In one series, demented patients showed an initial improvement and were able to maintain that improvement on continued doses of L-dopa for 5 months (25, 30). Examination of a wide range of cognitive assessments in another group of demented patients, however, failed to demonstrate any effect attributable to L-dopa (26).

Another important effect of L-dopa administration is the demonstration that mice treated with large doses of L-dopa have an increased life span (12, 13). Mice treated with high doses of L-dopa also retained a "youthful" appearance relative to controls (12, 13). Although Cotzias et al. (12, 13) did not find an effect of L-dopa on fertility, another investigator has noted an induction of ovulation in older female mice treated with L-dopa (29). Furthermore, this induction of ovulation was precipitated by administration of iproniazid (MAO inhibitor) or progesterone with equal efficacy. Hence, the animal model for a postmenopausal state demonstrates that ovulation can be induced potentially by either replacement hormone or inhibition of MAO activity.

SUMMARY

A number of pieces of evidence, not without controversy, converge to suggest that there is altered monoaminergic function in old age. In general, increases in monoamine oxidase in both central nervous system and some peripheral tissue and consistent decrements in monoamine content are correlated with advancing age. Further, strategies to reduce the increments in monoamine oxidase activity may be associated with reversals or cessations of some aging processes. The lack of consistency in these data requires further replication and pursuit in human populations in which altered monoaminergic function has been observed.

REFERENCES AND BIBLIOGRAPHY

1. Adolfsson R, Gottfries C, Roos B, Winblad B (1978): Postmortem analysis of monoamines and monoamine metabolites in brains from patients with senile dementia. Lakartaningen 75:650–652.

2. Aldinio C, Cerletti C, Manara L (1979): Human platelet monoamine oxidase activity in glaucoma. Invest Ophthalmol Vis Sci 18:320–324.

3. Aslan A (1956): A new method for prophylaxis and treatment of aging and Procaine-eutrophic and rejuvenating effects. Therapiewoche 7:14.

4. Aslan A (1974): Theoretical and practice aspects of chemotherapeutic techniques in the retardation of the aging process. In Rockstein M, ed: Theoretical Aspects of Aging. New York, Academic Press, pp 145–156.

5. Axelrod J (1959): Metabolism of epinephrine and other sympathomimetic amines. Physiol Rev 39:751.

6. Bridge TP, Potkin SG, Wise CD, Wyatt RJ (1979): Older schizophrenics: Symptomatology and platelet monoamine oxidase. Presented at 32nd Annual Meetings of the Gerontological Society, Washington, DC.

7. Bridge TP, Wise CD, Potkin SG, Phelps BH, Wyatt RJ (1979): Platelet monoamine oxidase: Studies of activity and thermolability in a general population. Presented at the ACNP Meeting, December.

8. Brockington I, Crow TJ, Johnstone EC, Owen F (1976) An investigation of platelet monoamine oxidase activity in schizophrenia and schizoaffective psychoses. In: CIBA Foundation Symposium 39: Monoamine Oxidase and Its Inhibition. Amsterdam, Elsevier.

9. Carlsson A, Winblad A (1976): Influence of age and time interval between death and autopsy on dopamine and 3 methoxytyramine levels in human basal ganglia. J Neural Transm 38:271–276.

10. Cohen S, Ditman K (1974): Gerovital H_3 in the treatment of the depressed aging patient. Psychosomatics 15:15–19.

11. Cohen DJ, Young JL, Roth JA (1977): Platelet monoamine oxidase in early childhood autism. Arch Gen Psychiatry 34:534–537.

12. Cotzias, GC, Miller ST, Nicholson AR, Maston WH, Tang LC (1974): Prologation of the life span in mice adapted to large amounts of L-DOPA. Proc Natl Acad Sci 71:2466–2469.

13. Cotzias GC, Miller ST, Tang LC, Papavasiliou PS (1977): Levodopa, fertility and longevity. Science 196:549–551.

14. Diamond SG, Markham CH (1976): Present mortality in Parkinson's disease: The ratio of observed to expected deaths with a method to calculate expected deaths. J Neural Transm 38:259–269.

15. Diez A, Maderdrut JL (1977): Development of multiple forms of mouse brain monoamine oxidase *in vivo* and *in vitro*. Brain Res 128:187–192.

16. Feldman J, Roche JM (1978): Effects of aging on monoamine oxidase activity of mouse and rabbit tissue. Exp Aging Res 4:97–107.

17. Fuentes JA, Trepel JB, Neff NH (1977): Monoamine oxidase activity in the cardiovascular system of young and aged rats. Exp Gerontol 12:113–115.

18. Fuller RN, Rouse BW (1977): Procaine hydrochloride as a monoamine oxidase inhibitor: Implications for geriatric therapy. J Am Geriatr Soc 25:90–93.

19. Gandhi BS, Kanungo MS (1974): Effects of cortisone on monoamine oxidase of the liver of young and old rats. Indian J Biochem Biophys 11:102–104.

20. Gershon ES, Belmaker RH, Ebstein R, Jonas WZ (1977): Plasma monoamine activity unrelated to genetic vulnerability to primary affective illness. Arch Gen Psychiatry 34:731–734.

21. Gey KF, Burkhead WP, Peltscher A. Variation of the norepinephrine metabolism of the rat heart with age. Gerontologica 11:1.

22. Gripois D (1975): Development characteristics of monoamine oxidase, Comp Biochem Physiol 51:143–151.

23. Horita A (1968): The influence of age on the recovery of cardiac monoamine oxidase after irreversible inhibition. Biochem Pharmacol 17:2091.

24. Horita A, Lowe MC. On the extra neuronal nature of cardiac monoamine oxidase in the rat. In Costa E, Sander M, eds: Monoamine Oxidase: New Vistas, New York, Raven Press, pp 227–242.

25. Johnson K, Presler AS, Ballinger BR (1978): Levodopa in senile dementia, Br Med J 1:1625.

26. Kristensen V, Olsen M, Thielgard A (1976): Levodopa treatment of presenile dementia. Acta Psychiatr Scand. 55:41–51.

27. Lai FM, Berkowitz B, Spector J (1978): Influence of age on brain vascular and cardiovascular monoamine oxidase activity in the rat. Life Sci 22:2051–2056.

28. Lees AJ, Shaw M, Kohout LJ (1977): Deprenyl in Parkinson's disease. Lancet 2:791–795.

29. Lehman JR, McArthur DA, Hendricks SE (1978): Pharmacological induction on ovulation in old and neonatally androgenized rats. Exp Gerontol 13:107–114.

30. Lewis C, Ballinger BR, Presler AJ (1978): Trial of levodopa in senile dementia. Br Med J 1:550.

31. McFarlane MD (1973): Possible rationale for procaine (Gerovital H_3) therapy in geriatrics: Inhibition of monoamine oxidase, J Am Geriatr Soc 21:414–418.

32. McFarlane MD, Besbris H (1974): Procaine (Gerovital H_3) therapy: Mechanism of inhibition of monoamine oxidase. J Am Geriat Soc 22:365–371.

33. Murphy DL, Belmaker R, Wyatt RJ (1974): Monoamine oxidase in schizophrenia and other behavioral disorders. J Psychiatry Res 11:221–247.

34. Murphy DL, Redmond DE, Bueller J, Donnelly CH (1978): Platelet monoamine oxidase activity in 116 normal rhesus monkeys, Comp Biochem Physiol 60:105–108.

35. Murphy DL, Weiss R (1972): Reduced monoamine oxidase activity in blood and platelets from bipolar depressed patients. Am J Psychiatry 128:1351–1357.

36. Natatsu T, Kato S, Sano M (1977): Tyrosine hydroxylase and DOPA decarboxylase activities and neuropathologic findings in brain regions of Parkinson patients. Adv Neurol Sci 21:441–446.

37. Nies A, Robinson DS, Davis JM, Ravaris A (1973): Changes in monoamines oxidase with aging. In Eisendorfer C, Fann WE, eds: Psychopharmacology and Aging, New York, Plenum Press, pp 41–53.

38. Novick WS (1961): The effect of age and thyroid hormones on the monoamine oxidase of rat heart. Endocrinology 69:55–59.

39. Officer JE (1974): Procaine-HCL growth enhancing effects on aged mouse embryo fibroblasts cultured in vitro. In Rockstein M, ed: Theoretical Aspects of Aging, New York, Academic Press, pp 167–175.

40. Olsen EJ, Banh L, Jarvik LF (1978): Gerovital H_3: A clinical trial as an antidepressant. J Gerontol 33:514–520.

41. Orsulak PJ, Schildkraut JJ, Schatzberg AF, Herzog JM (1978): Differences in platelet monoamine oxidase in subgroups of schizophrenic and depressive disorders. Biol Psychiatry 13:637–647.

42. Owen F, Cross AJ, Lofthouse R (1979): Distribution and inhibition of human brain monoamine oxidase. Biochem Pharmacol 28:1077–1080.

43. Prange AJ, White JE, Lipton MA, Kinkead MA (1967): Influence of age on monoamine oxidase and catechol-o-methyl transferase in rat tissues. Life Sci 6:581–586.

44. Radha E (1978): Age related responsiveness of monoamine oxidase inhibitors. Adv Exp Med Biol 108:301–308.

45. Robinson DS (1974): Changes in monoamine oxidase and monoamines with human development and aging. Fed Proc 34:103–107.

46. Robinson DS, Davis JM, Nies A, Bunney WE, Davis JM, Colburn RN, Bourne HR, Shaw DM, Coppen AJ (1972): Ageing, monoamines, and monoamine oxidase levels. Lancet 1:290.

47. Robinson DS, Davis JM, Nies A, Ravaris CL, Sylvester D (1971): Relation of sex and aging to monoamine oxidase activity of human brain, plasma, and platelets. Arch Gen Psychiatry 24:536–539.

48. Shih JC (1975): Multiple forms of monoamine oxidase and aging. In Brody H, Harman D, Ordy JM, eds: Aging, Vol. II. New York, Raven Press, pp 191–198.

49. Simpkins JW, Mueller GP, Huang HH, Meites J (1977): Evidence for depressed catecholamine and enhanced serotonin in aging male rats. Endocrinology 100: 1672–1685.

50. Takahashi S (1977): Monoamine oxidase activity in blood platelets from manic and depressed patients. Fol Neurol Japan 31:37–48.

51. VonKnooring L, Oreland L, Perris C (1977): Neurophysiological measures and visual averaged evoked responses in psychiatric patients. Neuropsychobiology 3:65–74.

52. Winblad B, Adolfsson R, Aquilonius SM, Eckerhaus SA, Gottfries CG, Oreland L, Wiberg A (1978): Monoaminergic activity in old age and patients with dementia disorders of the Alzheimer type. In: Report of II World Congress of Biologic Psychiatry, Barcelona.

53. Winblad B, Gottfries C, Oreland L, Wiberg A (1979): Monoamine oxidase in platelets and brains of non psychiatric and non neurological geriatric patients. Med Biol 57:129–132.

54. Ziegler MG, Lake CR, Kopin IJ (1976): Plasma noradrenalin increases with age. Nature 261:333–335.

55. Zung WW, Gianturco D, Pfeiffer E, Wang HS, Bridge TP, Potkin SG (1974): Pharmacology of depression in the aged: Evaluation of gerovital H_3 as an antidepressant drug. Psychosomatics 15:127–131.

II

CLINICAL IMPLICATIONS
FOR PSYCHOACTIVE DRUG USE

7

POTENTIAL DRUG INTERACTIONS IN AGING PATIENTS

Terrence F. Blaschke

Man may escape from rope and gun;
Nay, some have out-lived the Doctors pill.

John Gay (1685–1732), *The Beggars' Opera*

The growing number of reported drug–drug interactions and the absence of good epidemiologic evidence of the incidence of adverse reactions due to drug interactions have resulted in confusion and skepticism about their clinical importance. A number of recent review articles have attempted to put this topic into perspective (2, 3, 10, 24, 25). The basic problem, however, is an inadequate base of information from which to judge the medical, social, and economic effects of drug–drug interactions (1).

The use of more than one drug concurrently in the same patient is often necessary for optimal care. However, the use of multiple drug therapy places a responsibility on the physician to be alert to the possibility that drug interactions may occur. Only a subset of drug combinations have the potential to interact, and, of that subset, only a small fraction of the interactions result in adverse drug reactions (15, 25, 31). Much of the uncertainty about drug interactions relates to this gap between the frequency with which patients receive potentially interacting combinations

From the Division of Clinical Pharmacology, Stanford University School of Medicine, Stanford, California 94305.

Supported in part by USPHS grants AG01340 and HS00739. Terrence F. Blaschke is a Burroughs Wellcome Scholar in Clinical Pharmacology and the recipient of a RCDA (GM00407) from the NIH as compared to the incidence of negative drug interactions. This discrepancy is compounded by the use of various data bases for identifying potentially interacting combinations of drugs. Those that include animal in vitro or case report data result in a greater frequency of potential interactions, while those that include only those interactions known to produce adverse affects in a significant proportion of patients will result in a low frequency. The former type of data base might "desensitize" physicians to the extent that they fail to consider drug interactions as a cause of therapeutic problems, while the latter type might not alert them to patients at risk of an adverse drug reaction caused by less common drug interactions.

A number of factors contribute to the propensity for developing a negative drug interaction. Age has been cited as one of those factors (22, 35) but age per se may be less important than other factors that are more common in aging patients than in younger patients. This chapter reviews some of the age-dependent factors that can affect the incidence of adverse drug interactions and will present data concerning the frequency with which potentially interacting drug combinations are prescribed for elderly patients. The frequent use of psychoactive drugs in this age group (41, 42) and their frequent interaction with many drugs (7, 39) results in a high potential for adverse drug reactions.

THE DRUG INTERACTION INFORMATION PROBLEM

The therapist faces two specific problems when administering more than one drug to the same patient. One is remembering whether a specific combination has the potential to result in an interaction (by any of several mechanisms). The second is determining what action is necessary to avoid the adverse consequences of the interaction or to take advantage of the interaction to increase efficacy (e.g., with antihypertensive agents). While many physicians are aware of some important potential drug–drug interactions, the results of several epidemiologic studies indicate that both well-known and less familiar drug interactions go undetected and lead to unwanted effects (18, 21). This consequence is related to the magnitude of the information problem for drug interactions, which makes it likely that even physicians who are both well informed and careful will overlook important interactions.

As the number of prescriptions given at the same time to the same patient increases there is a sharp increase in the number of possible combinations which must be considered in terms of their potential to interact. The general expression for the number of different combinations of two drugs for a given set of drugs is

$$\text{number of combinations} =$$
$$\text{(number of drugs)!}/[2! \text{ (number of drugs} - 2)!]$$

Thus, if a patient is receiving seven drugs concurrently, there are 21 different possible combinations of two drugs, and if a patient is receiving 10 drugs concurrently, there are 45 different combinations of two drugs. Coadministration of more than one drug to the same patient is very common, especially in the inpatient or nursing home setting. In surveys carried out at a series of nursing homes there was an average of 3.2 to 7.7 prescriptions per nursing home patient (8, 12, 36, 39) and the Task Force on Prescription Drugs (41, 42) found that patients over age 45 fill an average of almost 14 prescriptions each year. At acute care hospitals and on general medical services, it is not unusual to find that 10% or more of patients are receiving more than 10 drugs simultaneously. Clearly the magnitude of the monitoring problem is substantial, increasing the likelihood of oversights and lending itself to automated monitoring approaches (11, 15).

DRUG INTERACTIONS AND ADVERSE DRUG REACTIONS

The term "drug interaction" is not synonymous with "contraindicated combination." The fact that two or more drugs have the potential to interact does not usually require discontinuation of a drug, but it may necessitate a change in dose, route, or frequency or additional clinical or laboratory monitoring of the patient. Some interactions lead to desirable effects (such as the use of probenecid with penicillin), but most of the attention has focused on drug interactions that lead to increased morbidity and mortality. The unanswered critical question is how often drug–drug interactions result in adverse drug reactions (1). The Boston Collaborative Drug Surveillance Program (BCDSP) estimated that approximately 22% of adverse drug reactions are related to drug–drug interactions (6). However, the BCDSP provides scanty information on the criteria used to define an adverse drug reaction and no information on the clinical significance and severity of the adverse drug reaction. Most of the available literature on the adverse consequences of drug–drug interactions is of the case report variety and provides no data concerning the magnitude, clinical significance, and economic consequences of this problem. In a recent study, May et al. (29) observed an increased incidence of adverse reactions to nine index drugs in patients who were receiving greater numbers of other drugs. While such data suggest that drug interactions during multiple drug therapy may result in an increased incidence of adverse reaction, these data are also open to other interpretations, including the possibility that sicker patients are more likely to receive more drugs and, because of more serious underlying disease, are more likely to have adverse reactions to a drug in the index group even when it is given alone.

Several investigators have studied and documented the considerable difficulties in obtaining valid information about the frequency and importance of adverse drug reactions, which also applies to drug reactions related to drug interactions (5, 24, 26). A problem rarely considered in discussing the clinical incidence and significance of adverse drug reactions is that most reactions are defined in terms of the development of toxic symptoms and are identified only if toxicity occurs. Many drug interactions, such as those involving enzyme-inducing agents or those interfering with absorption, do not lead to drug toxicity but instead result in a loss of efficacy. Interactions of this type are extremely difficult to detect, since they are often mistaken for disease progression or therapeutic failure (28). These interactions also represent adverse consequences due to drug interactions. They will be detected, however, only when the physician has a high index of suspicion (30).

A working knowledge of the various mechanisms by which drug interactions occur is of value in detecting possible interactions (Table 1) and reduces the need to memorize large lists. A familiarity with mechanisms provides a logical framework in which to consider drug interactions and fosters the transference of information to clinical settings. Several excellent reviews of mechanisms and of specific interactions are available, including Cohen and Armstrong (10), Hansten (20), and Morrelli and Melmon (33).

TABLE 1. Mechanisms of Drug–Drug Interactions

Category	Example
A. Pharmaceutical incompatibility, i.e., direct chemical–chemical or chemical–container interactions	Cephalothin–gentamicin
B. Pharmacokinetic interactions	
1. Altered rate or extent of absorption	Tetracycline–ferrous sulfate
2. Changes in binding by plasma proteins or tissues and/or the extent of distribution	Clofibrate–warfarin (complex mechanism)
3. Altered drug metabolism	
induction of drug metabolizing enzymes	Rifampicin–warfarin
inhibition of drug metabolizing enzymes	Chloramphenicol–phenytoin
4. Changes in renal excretion (increased/decreased filtration, secretion, reabsorption)	Probenecid–penicillin
C. Interactions at the receptor site	Guanethidine–desipramine
D. Additive pharmacologic effects	Potassium chloride–spironolactone

SPECIAL CONSIDERATIONS IN THE AGING PATIENT

Despite methodologic problems, the few studies that have been done provide at least some support for the clinical impression that negative drug interactions are more common in the elderly (9, 22, 27, 35). The well-documented physiologic changes that occur with increasing age and the differences in physician prescribing habits for the aging patient lend theoretical support to the notion that this population is at greater risk for adverse drug reactions. These physiologic and drug use factors are summarized in Table 2.

The physiologic consequences of aging on body composition, serum proteins, renal function, and hepatic metabolism have been reviewed elsewhere (37) (see also Chapters 1 and 3). These changes are of sufficient magnitude to cause substantial differences in the disposition of many drugs in otherwise healthy aging patients (13, 16, 46, 48) and, if adjustments in dose are not made, may result in a higher incidence of adverse drug reactions to individual drugs. When drug combinations are administered, pharmacokinetic interactions are more likely to result in toxicity, because the pharmacologic response to individual components may be greater than observed in younger patients (4).

Altered tissue distribution and plasma protein binding of some drugs have been reported in elderly patients. These differences make elderly patients more susceptible to displacement interactions, and decrease the utility of drug concentration measurements in plasma or serum as a guide to therapeutic monitoring. Alterations in receptor "sensitivity" have also been postulated to exist in elderly patients. Recent data obtained for propranolol seem to confirm an apparent decrease in sensitivity to beta receptors in elderly patients (47). Shepherd and coworkers (40) have

TABLE 2. **Factors Predisposing to Drug Interactions in Aging Patients**

Physiologic factors
  Decreased renal function
  Impaired drug metabolism
  Altered tissue distribution/binding
  Increased receptor "sensitivity"
  Diminished compensatory reflexes

Prescribing habits
  Use of "standard" doses of drugs
  Long-term use of many drugs with narrow therapeutic ratios (glycosides, antiarrhythmics)
  Multiple sources of drugs (e.g., gynecologist, internist, surgeon, ear–nose–throat, etc.)
  Use of over the counter preparations
  Lack of awareness of unintended pharmacologic actions of drugs

reported on increased sensitivity to warfarin in aging patients. The mechanisms of such changes in sensitivity are not clear at present. However, they could lead to a higher incidence of negative drug interactions. Much more work is needed to establish the extent and relevance of these preliminary studies of receptor differences due to aging, differences that may eventually account for much of the observed clinical variability in response between young and old patients.

An important, but frequently overlooked, factor that influences drug response in the elderly is the impairment of homeostatic control systems. Thus, the fall in blood pressure produced by two drugs that decrease peripheral resistance is likely to provoke an increased heart rate in young subjects to maintain cerebral perfusion, whereas the heart rate of the aging patient may not respond as well, and serious hypotension may occur (23). Similarly, the response to hypoglycemia produced by a drug interaction may be blunted in the aging patient. This inadequacy of homeostatic responses greatly increases the likelihood that a drug interaction that would be insignificant in a younger patient will assume clinical importance in an elderly patient (48).

Differences in the use of drugs by the elderly due to both physician and patient habits are another reason a greater incidence of adverse consequences caused by drug interactions might be anticipated in elderly patients. An easily identifiable and correctable problem is the use of "standard" doses of concurrently administered drugs in the elderly patient. Adult dosages, which are found in the common sources of prescribing information (e.g., the *Physician's Desk Reference*), are usually derived from studies in younger patients and may not take into account the decreased renal and metabolic function mentioned earlier. Drug treatment in elderly patients also tends to be more chronic in duration, and the types of drugs used most frequently (glycosides, antihypertensives, neuroleptics, and antiarrhythmics) tend to have a narrow therapeutic ratio. The aging patient often has multiple sources of drug therapy, especially when care is divided among a variety of subspecialists. These patients also tend to take more over-the-counter preparations because of an increased frequency of sleep disturbances and somatic symptoms. Finally, there may be a lack of awareness on the part of the physician of unintended pharmacologic actions of drugs that can lead to adverse drug reactions in the elderly because of impaired homeostatic responses.

These differences in physiology and drug use between young and old patients can account for a large part of the observed increase in adverse drug reaction, and, presumably, negative drug interactions found in epidemiologic studies (19, 22, 34, 39). The additional finding that there appears to be a higher frequency of potential drug–drug interactions in hospitalized or institutionalized aging patients (8, 12) is further evidence that they contribute significantly to iatrogenic morbidity and mortality in this population. However, as mentioned previously, documentation of the precise magnitude of the drug interaction/adverse drug reaction problem has not been done and would require a large scale intensive monitoring approach. Although difficult to obtain, such information is critical in assessing the cost/benefit ratio of interaction monitoring systems and in designing specific educational programs related to drug interaction programs (1).

AGING AND INTERACTIONS INVOLVING PSYCHOACTIVE DRUGS

Drugs acting on the central nervous system are the most common type of drugs prescribed for patients over age 65 (39, 41, 42). It is hardly surprising, therefore, that they are involved in a large fraction of potential drug interactions seen when monitoring is carried out (14). In a study of seven nursing homes, for example, Cooper and coworkers (12) showed that, excluding digitalis/diuretic interactions, half of the remaining potential interactions involved centrally active drugs.

At Stanford, a computer-based system (32, 43, 44, 45) has been used to determine the number of potential drug interactions in 1965 patients receiving drugs in nursing home settings. Monitored patients received an average of six drugs, and about 20% of the patients received a potentially interacting drug combination. In contrast to the latter figure, only 1 in 15 new prescriptions results in a potential interaction. This distinction is of some importance to the problem of physician monitoring, because it illustrates that while one of every five patients is at risk of an adverse drug reaction due to a drug interaction, the prescriber must consider 15 combinations to identify 1 with the potential to interact. Additionally, the data show that 10% of these patients were receiving 12 or more drugs, which is surprising in view of the fact that these are nonacute care patients residing in nursing homes.

Table 3 lists the 25 most frequent potential drug interactions in the Stanford nursing home survey, according to the carefully documented data base of this system (10). The frequency of a particular interaction on this list is different from that observed by other epidemiologic studies at Stanford or other acute care hospitals (6, 29) because of differences in the therapeutic categories of drugs used in acute, as compared to chronic, facilities. Nearly half the 25 interactions listed involve psychoactive drugs, and they represent nearly half the total number of potential interactions as well. The interactions listed in Table 3 vary widely in terms of how often an adverse consequence might result from a particular drug combination and in terms of the severity of a potential interaction (18). Some, such as those involving potassium preparations and potassium-sparing diuretics, have been documented to result in a high proportion of serious adverse drug reactions. Some potential drug interactions that may be reasonably

TABLE 3. Twenty-five Most Frequently Prescribed Potential Drug Interactions

Potentially interacting combinations	
Aluminum adsorbents	Phenothiazines—oral
Corticosteroids	Salicylates
D vitamins	Thiazide diuretics
Anticholinergic drugs	Phenothiazines—oral
Barbiturates	Corticosteroids
Salicylates	Sulfonylureas
Phenothiazines	Tricyclic antidepressants
Furosemide	Sulfonylureas
Barbiturates	Tricyclic antidepressants
Folic acid	Hydantoins
A vitamins	Mineral oil
Sympathomimetic amines	Tricyclic antidepressants
Corticosteroids	Hydantoins
Ethanol-1	Salicylates
Ethanol-1	Phenothiazines
Salicylates	Spironolactone
Potassium preparations	Triamterene
Aminoglycoside antibiotics	Polypeptide antibiotics
Alphamethyldopa	Sympathomimetic amines
Sulfonylureas	Thiazide diuretics
Potassium preparations	Spironolactone
Levodopa	Pyridoxine
Barbiturates	Ethanol-1
Digitalis preparations	Thiazide diuretics
Thyroid hormones	Tricyclic antidepressants

frequent but are not included on this list are absorption interactions involving antacids and benzodiazepines (17), which result in slower absorption but no change in the extent of absorption. This type of interaction (delayed absorption) may be of clinical significance when diazepam is used in a single-dose setting, such as for acute anxiety or sedation. For a thorough discussion of each of the interactions listed in Table 3, including primary literature documentation, the reader is referred to Hansten (20) and Cohen and Armstrong (10).

The overall frequency of potential drug interactions shown in Table 3 is lower than that from other published data (8, 12, 31, 39) primarily because a more rigorous data base is used. Although 20% of elderly institutionalized patients are exposed to the risk of an adverse drug reaction due to drug interactions, these figures cannot and should not be extrapolated to the aging population at large. The types of potential interactions seen are consistent with data concerning drug use studies in aging patients (39, 42, 48). However, there are still no data to determine whether the incidence of adverse clinical effects of drug–drug interactions is higher in old than in young patients receiving two or more drugs. Nevertheless, as can be seen in Table 2, changes in physiologic function of the liver and kidneys, changes in cardiovascular reserve, alterations in body composition, differences in plasma and tissue drug binding, and increases in receptor sensitivity put the aging patient at much greater risk of an adverse drug reaction from a drug given alone or drugs given in combination.

It might be tempting to conclude that the problem of adverse drug reactions in aging patients could be limited by reducing drug use in this population. Few, if any, of the drug combinations listed in Table 3 can a priori be considered irrational, and all may be appropriate for a given clinical setting. It is certainly desirable to avoid multiple drug therapy in any patient, young or old; however, this should not be practiced at the expense of withholding drugs that may improve the quantity or quality of life. The therapist has the responsibility to use drugs optimally in aging patients, which requires a knowledge of the very real differences in dosages that exist for many drugs owing to changes in drug disposition or sensitivity. When prescribing a rational combination of drugs to an older patient, the physician must be aware of potential drug interactions, must adjust doses accordingly, and must maintain a high level of vigilance (often necessitating closer laboratory follow-up) during the course of treatment with drug combinations. In this way, each patient will receive optimal treatment.

I would like to thank the staff of the MEDIPHOR project for their assistance in compiling the interaction data and Linda Halloran for preparing the manuscript.

REFERENCES AND BIBLIOGRAPHY

1. Adverse Drug Reactions in the United States: An Analysis of the Scope of the Problem and Recommendations for Future Approaches (1974): Medicine in the Public Interest. Washington, DC.

2. Avery GS (1977): Drug interactions that really matter: A guide to major important drug interactions. Drugs 14:132–146.

3. Azarnoff DL (1974): Drug interactions: Clinical significance. Clin Pharmacol Ther 16:986–988.

4. Bender AD (1974): Pharmacodynamic principles of drug therapy in the aged. J Am Geriatr Soc 22:296–303.

5. Blanc S, Leuenberger P, Berger J-P, Brooke EM, Schelling J-L (1979): Judgements of trained observers on adverse drug reactions. Clin Pharmacol Ther 25:493–498.

6. Borda IT, Slone D, Jick H (1968): Assessment of adverse reactions within a drug surveillance program. JAMA 205:99–101.

7. Braithwaite RA (1976): The significance of drug interactions in the evaluation of psychotropic drugs. Br J Clin Pharmacol (Suppl 1) 3:29–34.

8. Brown MM, Boosinger JK, Henderson M, Rife SS, Rustia JK, Taylor O, Young WW (1977): Drug–drug interactions among residents in homes for the elderly: A pilot study. Nurs Res 26:47–52.

9. Cadwallader DE (1979): Drug interactions in the elderly. In Peterson DM, Whittington FJ, Payne BP, eds: Drugs and the Elderly. Springfield, Ill, Thomas, pp 80–93.
10. Cohen SN, Armstrong MF (1974): Drug Interactions. A Handbook for Clinical Use. Baltimore, Williams & Wilkins.
11. Cohen SN, Armstrong, MF, Briggs RL, et al. (1974): A computer-based system for the study and control of drug interactions in hospitalized patients. In Morselli PL, Garattini S, Cohen SN, eds: New York, Raven Press, pp 363–374.
12. Cooper JW, Wellins I, Fish KH, Loomis ME (1975): Frequency of potential drug–drug interactions: A seven nursing home study. J Am Pharmaceut Assoc 15:24–31, 1975.
13. Crooks J, O'Malley K, Stevenson IH (1976): Pharmacokinetics in the elderly. Clin Pharmacokinet, 1:280–296.
14. Fann WE (1973): Interaction of psychotropic drugs in the elderly. Postgrad Med 53: 182–186.
15. Ford DR, Rivers NP, Wood GC (1977): A computerized detection system for potentially significant adverse drug–drug interactions. J Am Pharmaceut Assoc 17:354–357.
16. Garrod JW (1974): Absorption, metabolism and excretion of drugs in geriatric subjects. Gerontol Clin 16:30–42.
17. Greenblatt DJ, Allen MD, MacLaughlin DS, Harmatz JS, Shader RI (1978): Diazepam absorption: Effects of antacids and food. Clin Pharmacol Ther 24:600–609.
18. Greenblatt DJ, Koch-Weser J (1973): Adverse reactions to spironolactone JAMA 225: 40–43.
19. Hall MRP (1974): Adverse drug reactions in the elderly. Geront Clin 166:144–150.
20. Hansten PD (1979): Drug Interactions, ed 4. Philadelphia, Lea & Febiger.
21. Hull JH, Murray WJ, Brown HS, Williams BO, Chi SL, Koch GG (1978): Potential anticoagulant drug interactions in ambulatory patients. Clin Pharmacol Ther 24:644–649.
22. Hurwitz N (1969): Predisposing factors in reactions to drugs. Br Med J 1:531–536.
23. Jackson G, Pierscianowski TA, Mahon W, Condon J (1976): Inappropriate antihypertensive therapy in the elderly. Lancet 2:1317–1318.
24. Karch FE, Lasagna L (1975): Adverse drug reactions. A critical review JAMA 234: 1236–1241.
25. Koch-Weser J, Greenblatt DJ (1977): Drug interactions in clinical perspective. Eur J Clin Pharmacol 11:405–408.
26. Koch-Weser J, Sellers EM, Zacest R (1977): The ambiguity of adverse drug reactions. Eur J Clin Pharmacol 11:75–78.
27. Law R, Chalmers C (1976): Medicines and elderly people: A general practice survey. Br Med J 1:565–568.
28. MacLennan WJ (1974): Drug interactions. Gerontol Clin 16:18–24.
29. May FE, Stewart RB, Cluff LE (1977): Drug interactions and multiple drug administration. Clin Pharmacol Ther 22:322–328.
30. Melmon KL (1971): Preventable drug reactions—Causes and cures. N Engl J Med 284:1361–1368.
31. Mitchell GW, Stanazek WF, Nicholo NB (1979): Documenting drug–drug interactions in ambulatory patients. Am J Hosp Pharm 36:653–657.
32. Morrell J, Podlone M, Cohen SN (1977): Receptivity of physicians in a teaching hospital to a computerized drug interaction monitoring and reporting system. Med Care 15: 68–78.
33. Morrelli HF, Melmon KL (1978): Drug interactions. In Melmon KL, Morrelli HF, eds: Clinical Pharmacology: Basic Principles in Therapeutics. New York, Macmillan.
34. Peterson DM, Thomas CW (1975): Acute drug reactions among the elderly. J Gerontol 30:552–556.

35. Peterson DM, Whittington FJ, Payne BP, eds (1979): Drugs and the Elderly. Springfield, Ill, Thomas.

36. Rawlings JL, Frisk PA (1975): Pharmaceutical services for skilled nursing facilities in compliance with federal regulation. Am J Hosp Pharm 32:905–908.

37. Richey DP (1975): Effects of human aging on drug absorption and metabolism. In Goldman R, Rockstein M, eds: The Physiology and Pathology of Human Aging. New York, Academic Press, pp 59–93.

38. Rickey DP, Bender AD (1977): Pharmacokinetic consequences of aging. Annu Rev Pharmacol Toxicol 17:49–65.

39. Segal JL, Thompson JF, Floyd RA (1979): Drug use and prescribing patterns in a skilled nursing facility: The need for a rational approach to therapeutics. J Am Geriatr Soc 27:117–122.

40. Shepherd AMM, Hewick DS, Moreland TH, Stevenson IH (1977): Age as a determinant of sensitivity to warfarin. Br J Clin Pharmacol 4:315–320.

41. Task Force on Prescription Drugs (1968): The Drug Users. Washington, DC, US Department of Health Education and Welfare, US Government Printing Office.

42. Task Force on Prescription Drugs (1969): Final Report. Washington, DC, US Department of Health, Education and Welfare, US Government Printing Office.

43. Tatro DS (1975). Online drug interaction surveillance. Am J Hosp Pharm 32:417–422.

44. Tatro DS, Briggs RL, Chavez-Pardo R, Feinberg LS, Hannigan JF, Moore TN, Cohen SN (197). Detection and prevention of drug interactions utilizing an online computer system. Drug Info J 9:10–17.

45. Tatro DS, Moore TN, Cohen SN (1979): Computer-based system for adverse drug reaction detection and prevention. Am J Hosp Pharm 36:198–201.

46. Triggs EJ, Nation RL (1975): Pharmacokinetics in the aged: A review. J Pharmacokinet Biopharm 3:387–418.

47. Vestal RE, Wood AJJ, Shand DG (1979): Reduced beta adrenoceptor sensitivity in the elderly. Clin Pharmacol Ther 26:181–186.

48. Vestal RE (1978): Drug use in the elderly: A review of problems and special considerations. Drugs 16:358–382.

8

TRICYCLIC ANTIDEPRESSANTS AND CHILDREN

Judith L. Rapoport and William Z. Potter

The pediatric age group is a rich and varied clinical population in which to study the psychopharmacology of tricyclic antidepressants. This brief overview summarizes the four clinical conditions of childhood and adolescence in which tricyclics have been studied systematically: hyperkinesis, enuresis, school phobia, and most recently, depression. What little is known about plasma concentration, clinical and side effects, drug metabolism, and time course of clinical response is discussed, emphasizing the unique aspects of pharmacology of tricyclics for these age groups.

CLINICAL EFFICACY OF TRICYCLICS IN PEDIATRIC POPULATIONS

Two pediatric conditions have been shown to respond to tricyclic treatment at least on a short-term basis: enuresis and hyperkinesis. Reports on the treatment of these disorders (which represent all but two of the controlled studies with tricyclics in children) all indicate (1) an established immediate clinical effect often seen following the first dose, and (2) a wearing off of efficacy for many patients with chronic (2 to 5 week) drug administration.

In contrast, a few studies suggest a probable delayed effect of tricyclics with school-phobic and clinically depressed children.

Enuresis

Following the initial brief report of McLean (29) and a controlled clinical trial by Poussaint and Ditman (35), more than 30 double-blind studies

From the Unit on Childhood Mental Illness and the Clinical Psychobiology Branch, National Institute of Mental Health, and the National Institute of General Medical Sciences, Bethesda, Maryland.

A. Raskin, D. S. Robinson, and J. Levine, eds., Age and the Pharmacology of Psychoactive Drugs.

have demonstrated the symptomatic efficacy of tricyclic medication in enuresis (bedtime dosage from 25 to 125 mg).[1] While improvement is noted in 60 to 80% of most samples, total remissions are reported in only 10 to 50% during drug treatment for this condition, which has a significant placebo response rate. This literature has been reviewed extensively by Blackwell and Currah (1), who concluded that the case for cure of enuresis by tricyclics is not proved and that most children resume wetting when medication is stopped.

Most of the previous enuresis studies in children have not used either the same dose of tricyclic, similar populations or similar diagnostic criteria. For that reason, it has been difficult to make a statement about the comparative effectiveness of different tricyclics or to define "good responders" from the available reports. In general, institutionalized, retarded, and older enuretics and enuretics with daytime wetting seem to show a less favorable response.

In a recent study (26, 42) 20 disturbed and 20 nondisturbed severely enuretic boys were shown to respond equally well to both imipramine (IMI) and desmethylimipramine (DMI). The only significant predictor of clinical response was plasma concentration of the tricyclic, not behavioral disturbance in the child. However, the antienuretic response was not related simply to plasma level, because decreased effectiveness occurred in some children in spite of adequate plasma concentration of the drug. In the same study, the lack of effectiveness of methscopolamine indicates that peripheral anticholinergic mechanisms of action are not basic to anti-enuretic effect. Nonetheless, a central anticholinergic mechanism could still be operative.

Alternatively, the equivalence of DMI and IMI in the Rapoport et al. (42) study might indicate a noradrenergic antienuretic mechanism. Moreover, ephedrine, a sympathomimetic amine that activates alpha and beta receptors, reduced significantly the number of wet nights in a population of enuretics, although it was less effective than IMI (7). The lack of efficacy, however, of both methylphenidate and amphetamine (3, 8) might be used to argue against an adrenergic mode of action. It would be of great interest to compare the antienuretic effect of the presumed new antidepressants such as iprindol, mianserin, or zimelidine with imipramine, as an as yet unknown mechanism of tricyclics may be important in the treatment of enuresis. A recent comprehensive review of the physiology of micturition stresses the uncertain role of the sympathetic nervous system and the problems in interpreting pharmacologic results (46).

Hyperkinetic Behavior Disorders

Shortly after tricyclics began to be used for enuresis, reports on the use of the drugs in hyperactive/aggressive children claimed similar therapeutic

---

[1] The FDA maximum approved dose of imipramine for enuresis is 75 mg/day hs.

effects to those found with stimulants (19, 22, 39). More recently, controlled trials generally have confirmed these initial open studies and demonstrated the beneficial effect of tricyclics in doses from 2 to 5 mg/kg/day for restless, antisocial behavior (17, 25, 41, 52, 54). This response is immediate and in some cases dramatic; most of these studies, however, have shown methylphenidate or amphetamine to be superior to tricyclics.

All of these controlled studies are short term (4 weeks or less); the long-term usefulness of tricyclics for these disorders remains controversial. In an open study, Gittelman-Klein (10) indicated that an initial response observed at 2 weeks to a daily dose of 150 to 300 mg of IMI was not maintained at 12 weeks. Similarly, in a 1 year follow-up (38), significantly more hyperactive children had discontinued tricyclic medication than methylphenidate, even when both groups had shown an initial response after 6 weeks. It is our experience that long-term treatment of conduct-disordered or hyperkinetic children with tricyclics is unsatisfactory; this point deserves further study. In an unpublished study, attempts to predict IMI response in hyperactive children on the basis of clinical examination or history were unsuccessful (Rapoport and Quinn, unpublished data). For example, while about 25% of the sample of hyperactive boys showed some depressive symptomatology, this subgroup was not differentially responsive to tricyclic medication; also, a positive family history of depressive disorder was not predictive of response.

Separation Anxiety

A single double-blind study has shown that IMI benefits the separation anxiety associated with school phobia (11). This effect was seen after 6 weeks of treatment with an average daily dose of 152 mg. The authors stress that the anticipatory anxiety associated with school return did not seem altered. More studies are needed to confirm the usefulness of tricyclics in school phobics. Additionally, there are questions about their safety, since the doses said to be required are high and have been associated with one fatality. This study is of great interest, however, as it probably indicates a delayed effect (not seen at 3 weeks) in contrast to that seen with enuresis or hyperkinesis. This latter point is not completely certain, as the dose was increased over the 6 week period; thus dose-effect may be confounded with treatment duration.

Depressive Disorder

The difficulty in defining depressive disorder in childhood has been reviewed elsewhere and will not be discussed here (4, 15, 39, 40) except to note the apparent rarity of true adult-type depression in childhood and that the overuse of vague diagnostic labels such as "masked depression" or "depressive equivalent" has been detrimental to research in this area.

In controlled studies, IMI has been described as useful for a variety of possible depressive symptoms such as learning disabilities, irritability, dysphoria, insomnia, nightmares, and somatic manifestations (headaches and stomach aches) (24). Some of these studies (6, 27, 48) are particularly suggestive of true antidepressant action. These children, described as having social withdrawal, deteriorating school performance, and self-destruction of recent onset, seem to benefit from tricyclic medication. Most of these studies lack clear clinical description, objective behavior ratings, independent diagnostic ratings, or proper controls for time and placebo effects.

Puig-Antich et al. (36) have completed an open trial of IMI with eight children meeting the adult research diagnostic criteria (RDC) for depression (45). Behavior rating and clinical evaluation (using standardized scales) indicated that six of the eight improved on drug. This is the first methodologically adequate study of the antidepressant efficacy of a tricyclic in prepubertal children. Too few children have completed the double-blind protocol to form any conclusions; clinical response, however, appears to be delayed, occurring only after at least 2 weeks of treatment.

The interesting point here is that immediate clinical effects of tricyclics seen in children with hyperactivity or enuresis, conditions often regarded as "developmental delays," are probably mediated by a different mechanism than the delayed clinical effect seen after 2 to 4 weeks in depressed or school phobic children, i.e., those with "neurotic" disorders. These latter conditions are not associated with hyperactivity and enuresis and in fact occur more usually in children without signs of neurologic immaturity. This differing time course of drug effect may help validate these broad nosological categories. It may be that immediate effects of the drug, such as reuptake blockade of norepinephrine, are crucial for enuresis and hyperactivity, while alteration in receptor sensitivity is necessary for efficacy in school phobia or depression.

SIDE EFFECTS OF TRICYCLICS IN CHILDREN

DiMascio and Soltys (5) reviewed the antidepressant side-effect literature in children and found the incidence and severity of side effects to be generally similar to those reported in adults. Since that report, some specific questions of unique cardiovascular side effects of tricyclics in the pediatric age group have been raised. These will be discussed here.

Electrocardiograph

Winsberg et al. (53) reported electrocardiograph (ECG) changes in seven of seven children treated for hyperkinetic behavior disorders, receiving 5 mg/kg/day of IMI in divided doses. The principle changes were an increase in PR interval and a decrease in T wave magnitude, with an increase in width. There was no significant relationship of ECG changes to steady-state plasma concentration. These findings are similar to those reported for adults receiving IMI therapy (2, 23, 44). Saraf et al. (43) reviewed ECG changes in 33 children (8 school phobics and 25 hyper-actives) receiving between 4 and 5 mg/kg/day of IMI. They also reported increased pulse and PR intervals (although no T wave intervals). Although there were no data on plasma concentrations, there was a significant relationship between the dose and increase in PR interval, even when baseline PR interval (which also showed a relationship to drug effect) was partialed out. Further, there may be a positive relationship in children between mg/kg dose and plasma concentration of IMI. The clinical significance of these changes is uncertain however, as there may be differences between binding and metabolism of the tricyclics in children. It has also been speculated that children may be more susceptible to tricyclic induced cardiotoxicity than adults.

Cardiovascular

Five controlled systematic studies have shown an increase in blood pressure in children or young adolescents with tricyclic medication; these studies are listed in Table 1.

Rapoport et al. (41) compared imipramine, methylphenidate, and placebo treatments of hyperactive boys. Both IMI (mean dose 80 mg/day) and methylphenidate (30 mg/day) produced an elevation of diastolic blood pressure of 10 mm/Hg or more (31 and 26% in the treatment groups, respectively), while none of the placebo group showed this effect.

Greenberg and Yellin (16) reported similar increases in pulse and blood pressure, both systolic and diastolic, for 47 hyperactive children on IMI (100 mg/day) but not on methylphenidate or placebo. In the IMI group, three had an increase of 15 mm/Hg or more in diastolic blood pressure, requiring discontinuation of the drug.

Saraf et al. (43) reported a significant increase in mean standing diastolic BP for a group of 14 school phobic children and adolescents (from 72 to 81 mm/Hg; $p < .03$). Sitting pulse was also increased significantly.

Lake et al. (26) examined 14 children participating in a study of IMI treatment of enuresis with supine and standing blood pressure measurements. IMI (75 mg/hs) produced significant increases in pulse (supine and standing) and diastolic (but not systolic) blood pressure, both supine and standing. Plasma NE (supine, standing, and increment in NE with standing) were also increased, but this drug-related increase did not show any significant relationship with the pulse or blood pressure changes.

The effect on blood pressure, studied on the 13th treatment day in the Mikkelsen report, is the most complete analysis of tricyclic effects on blood pressure in children to date (supine and standing figures obtained for

TABLE 1. Imipramine: Effects on Blood Pressure in Pediatric Studies

	n	Age	Mean dose (IMI)	Duration	Sample	Results
Rapoport et al. (1974)	29 IMI 28 MP 19 Placebo	9 years	80 mg/day	6 weeks	Hyperactive	30% on IMI had diastolic BP increase ≥ 10 mm Hg 0% on placebo.
Werry et al. (1975)	24	8 years	50 mg/day	3 weeks	Enuretic	Increase in diastolic and systolic BP
Greenberg et al. (1975)	47	9 years	100 mg/day	5 weeks	Hyperactive	Increase in systolic and diastolic BP on IMI (not methylphenidate or placebo) (for 3 children ≥ 15 mm Hg)
Saraf et al. (1974)	14	10 years	132 mg/day	6 weeks	School phobic	Increase in standing diastolic BP (mean change from 72 mm Hg to 81 mm Hg) Systolic BP not increased
Mikkelsen et al. (1979)	14	9 years	75 mg/day	2 weeks	Enuretic	Increase in diastolic BP, supine and standing No significant change in systolic BP

IMI, imipramine   MP, methylphenidate

baseline, placebo, and drug condition). Plasma tricyclic concentration (IMI and DMI) correlated with the increase in diastolic blood pressure on drug ($r = .61$; $p < .03$).

In a clinical study with adult patients (ages not given), Blumberg et al. (2) found that schizophrenic adult patients showed a significant systolic BP increase, while depressed adult patients showed a systolic BP decrease on IMI (300 mg/day chronic treatment). Both diagnosis and age were significantly associated with this differential drug effect ($n = 39$; partial correlations: $-.31$ and $.43$, respectively). That is, younger patients and those who were schizophrenic were likely to get a blood pressure (BP) increase, while depressed and older patients were more likely to show a BP decrease on medication.

Similarly, Glassman et al. (12) found no effects of IMI on supine blood pressure in adult depressive patients, while standing BP revealed that the drug produced a significant and clinically noticeable fall in systolic pressure (13).

The relationship of these findings to those seen with children is not clear. In both groups, in spite of these different effects on diastolic blood pressure, orthostatic hypotension is a common side effect (21). A variety of children (school phobics and hyperactives) have been shown to have the diastolic BP increase, and it will be of interest to know whether the clinically depressed prepubertal patients of Puig-Antich et al. (37) show BP changes similar to adult depressives or to children with other disorders.

PHARMACOKINETICS OF TRICYCLICS IN CHILDREN

Plasma Concentration at Steady State

Little is known about the pharmacokinetics of tricyclic antidepressants in children, although preliminary reports have suggested that metabolism and protein binding are different than in adults (31, 50). Currently available clinical data are confined to the measurement of steady-state concentrations of IMI and its metabolites primarily in male children.

Pharmacokinetic studies can most simply reveal whether steady-state concentrations of tricyclics are similar after a specified milligram per kilogram dose to those observed in adults. Although a preliminary study suggested that children attain higher concentrations of IMI than adults (51), subsequent reports actually show that their IMI or IMI plus DMI concentrations are equivalent to or less than those found in adults (see Table 2). Neither Winsberg et al. (53), Puig-Antich et al. (37), nor Lake et al. (26) addressed the question of relative mean concentration of drug, so it was necessary to analyze their data retrospectively. In the case of the Lake et al. study, which included 40 boys (ages 7 to 12 years) treated with IMI for enuresis, the mean steady-state concentration of IMI plus DMI expressed as nanograms per milliliter per milligram per kilogram dose was

TABLE 2. Tricyclic Concentration in Children and Adults per Milligram per Kilogram Dose[a]

	Sum of IMI plus DMI concentration after IMI (ng/ml)	DMI concentration after DMI (ng/ml)[b]
Children		
Winsberg et al. (1975)		
$n = 7$	53	—
Rapoport et al. (1979)		
$n = 40$	52	48
Puig-Antich et al. (1979)		
$n = 13$	44	—
Adults		
Glassman et al. (1979)		
$n = 68$	57	—
Gram et al. (1977)		
$n = 76$	57	—
Potter et al. (1980)		
$n = 18$	62	44

[a]Observed concentration was divided by mg/kg of total daily administered dose. Concentrations are means from the referenced studies divided by either the given or estimated weights. For most studies, data for the calculation of mean ± standard deviation were not available.

[b]Steady-state concentrations of DMI following administration of DMI to either the same (42) or different patient population (33) reported for the IMI trial.

52 ng/ml. Puig-Antich et al. (36) in a sample of 13 children (aged 6 to 12 years) found a lower mean concentration of 44 ng/ml per mg/kg dose. If one asumes an average weight of 70 kg in the large reported adult sample of Glassman et al. (12), the mean IMI plus DMI concentration per milligram per kilogram dose is 57 ng/ml, and in the series reported by Gram et al. (15), in which concentrations were adjusted for dose, the finding is the same. A carefully monitored inpatient adult population achieved an IMI plus DMI concentration of 62 ng/ml per mg/kg dose (33).

A similar phenomenon is seen after DMI alone. In 20 boys aged 7 to 12 years, the mean steady-state DMI concentration was 48 ng/ml per mg/kg dose versus a concentration of 44 ng/ml per mg/kg in 10 adults (aged 22 to 67 years; 4 males, 6 females) (33, 34). Thus, children achieve concentrations of DMI or the sum of IMI plus DMI per milligram per kilogram dose similar to those found in adults.

This finding would not be apparent if one did not account for the milligram per kilogram dose. Plasma concentration of IMI or IMI plus all of its active metabolites following 75 mg/day dose is significantly correlated to weight in children (Figure 1), although this relationship only accounts for part of the variance in concentration ($r^2 = .32$ and .39, respectively). In

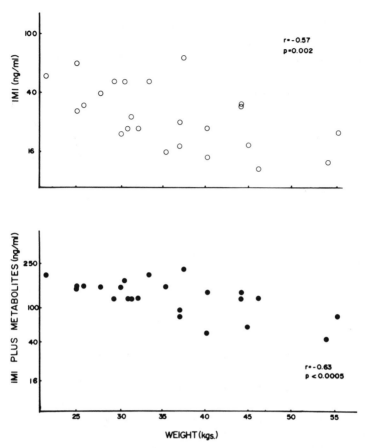

FIGURE 1. Relationship between concentration of imipramine (IMI) and IMI plus its active metabolites (OH-IMI, desipramine, and OH-desipramine) and weight in boys.

adults, presumably because the weight does not vary so dramatically, plasma concentration does not correlate with weight.

Therefore, on a milligram per kilogram basis, one might conclude that if toxicity is related to the mean steady-state concentration of IMI, DMI, or the sum of the two, IMI and DMI are as safe in children as in adults. A possible objection to this conclusion has been suggested by the observation that children (aged 3 to 14 years) have somewhat less protein binding of IMI than do adults (81.3 and 86.0%, respectively) (51). This difference is actually rather small and is even less for DMI (31); moreover, DMI is the form of drug that predominates in children after administration of IMI. In addition, these differences are based on an equilibrium dialysis technique that does not appear to give a true measure of bound drug (33) which, in the case of IMI and DMI, require conditions that do not interfere with binding to alpha-1-acid glycoprotein (32). Even if an age difference in binding were to be demonstrated, it would not affect the mean steady-state concentration of free IMI or DMI (i.e., that proportion of drug believed to be pharmacologically active).

This somewhat counterintuitive conclusion is based on more detailed pharmacokinetic discussions presented elsewhere (9). It may, however, be useful to briefly review the current understanding of the relationship between protein binding of drug, metabolism and steady-state concentration. Under steady-state conditions, following oral administration of a drug such as IMI which is cleared almost wholly by metabolism a simple equation may be used:

$$pC_{ss} = \text{dose}/Cl_{int}$$

where p is the fraction free in plasma (or whole blood), C_{ss} is the total (free and bound) steady-state concentration, dose is the maintenance dose (per 24 hours), and Cl_{int} is the intrinsic clearance or the maximal ability of the liver (and other sites) to metabolize the drug at zero blood flow.

pC_{ss} is the free steady-state concentration of drug and will, according to theory, be equal in all compartments (by definition at a true steady state). Since dose can be controlled and Cl_{int} is a given characteristic, the free concentration at steady-state for any one dose will be constant. If the fraction free increases, the total concentration (C_{ss}) will decrease. This phenomenon has been described in individuals who have decreased protein binding secondary to the nephrotic syndrome (18).

The more relevant and unstudied pharmacokinetic question in children is whether the peak and plasma concentration following either single or chronic IMI or DMI is different. Both altered volume of distribution and plasma protein binding of drug (which affects volume of distribution) will change the shape of the plasma concentration versus time curve although the total clearance or mean steady-state concentration will not be affected (8, 9). Thus, if either therapeutic effect or toxicity is best related to peak-plasma concentration, it would be helpful to know if there are major variations in volume of distribution or plasma protein binding in children or both. Unfortunately, even though it is known that IMI and DMI exert at least their antienuretic and antihyperkinetic effects almost immediately, no data relating peak concentration to effect are available. Furthermore, there do not appear to be any pharmacokinetic studies in children that allow for either accurate determinations of volume of distribution or plasma protein binding. If one were to accept the previously cited equilibrium dialysis data (51) as representative of the true range (if not the absolute amount of binding), the relatively small variation would indicate that alterations in protein binding are not likely to be significant clinically in children who suffer from enuresis, hyperkinesis, or depression in the absence of other pathology.

There is, however, another interesting phenomenon related to pharmacokinetics that is different in children and adults. In a preliminary report, it was suggested that following IMI children convert a greater proportion to DMI than do adults (51). This suggestion is given considerable experimental support in the report of Rapoport et al. (42) in 40 enuretic boys who report a mean IMI to DMI ratio of .54 (see Table 3) compared to a ratio of 1.1 in adults. Muscettola et al. (30) have shown that a greater proportion of DMI than of IMI is free in the cerebrospinal fluid of adults; extrapolating from this finding to our own results in children, one would predict that the IMI/DMI ratio in children would be .38 in the CSF. In other words, in children, one would expect DMI to be the predominant "active" moiety.

This may be oversimplifying the situation, since it is likely that hydroxylated metabolites of IMI are "active" psychoactive agents (33). It has been proposed that concentrations of hydroxyimipramine (OH-IMI) may be important for cardiotoxicity (20), although there are no clinical data to support this suggestion. Rather, in children following IMI there is very little OH-IMI but significant and presumably psychoactive concentrations of 2-hydroxydesipramine (OH-DMI). There is not, however, a marked difference in the ratio of OH-DMI to DMI in children, compared to adults (33).

In summary, three conclusions about IMI and DMI pharmacokinetics in children are possible on the basis of existing data: (1) Children clear IMI (demethylation to DMI) more rapidly than adults; (2) children clear the sum of IMI plus DMI after IMI, or DMI after DMI at a similar rate as do adults; and (3) hydroxylation of IMI and DMI in children and adults does not appear to be different. Although it is conceivable that there are clinically relevant differences in peak plasma concentrations between

TABLE 3. Plasma Tricyclic Concentration During Imipramine or Desmethylimipramine Treatment (ng/ml)

	Subject N	IMI Mean (SD)	DMI Mean (SD)	Total IMI plus DMI Mean (SD)	IMI/DMI ratio Mean (SD)
IMI Study phase	40	30.4 (± 17.6)	79.3 (±57.3)	109.3 (±56.2)	.54 (± .37)
DMI Study phase	20		98.3 (±65.7)		

children and adults (secondary to different volumes of distribution) no evidence is available to clarify this point.

Plasma Tricyclic Concentration and Clinical Efficacy

The reviewers were able to locate one partial report in a hyperactive group, a preliminary report in a depressed prepubertal group, and one report in an enuretic group.

Hyperactivity. Winsberg et al. (51) first presented data from a single case of a hyperactive boy for whom plasma tricyclic concentrations (IMI plus DMI) were followed serially along with classroom and ward observational data over an 11-day period. There seemed to be some relationship between the continued change in behavior and plasma concentration over time. However the authors stress (as noted previously) that the clinical effects of tricyclics are immediate, within 1 to 2 hours of the initial dose, and detailed studies of single dose pharmacokinetics have not been reported in children.

Winsberg et al. (51) reported a wide range of values (from 50 to 500 ng/ml) in children receiving the same per weight dose. One study of seven hospitalized aggressive prepubertal boys indicated that clinical improvement (i.e., decreased deviant behavior on the ward and increased

FIGURE 2. Relationship between plasma imipramine plus desmethylimipramine concentration in clinical antienuretic response.

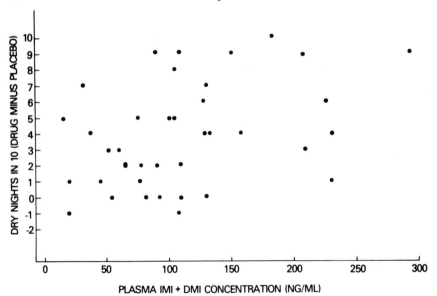

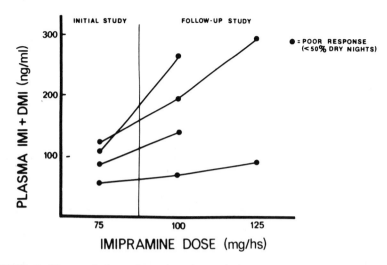

FIGURE 3. Plasma imipramine plus desmethylimipramine concentration and clinical follow-up for poor responders.

attentiveness in the hospital school) correlated with plasma tricyclic concentration (Winsberg et al., personal communication). This communication is regarded as preliminary by the authors.

Although no evidence is available, plasma concentrations would be of interest in chronic treatment of hyperactive children who demonstrate the

FIGURE 4. Plasma imipramine plus desmethylimipramine concentration and clinical follow-up for transient responders.

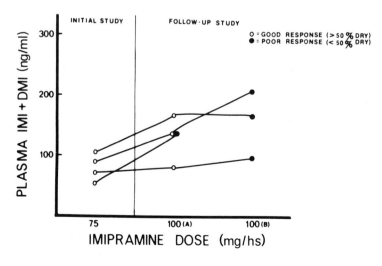

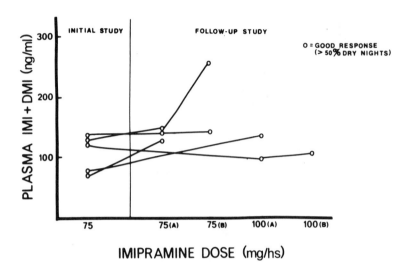

IMIPRAMINE DOSE (mg/hs)

FIGURE 5. Plasma imipramine plus desmethylimipramine concentration and clinical follow-up for good responders.

"wearoff" of clinical effect. If sustained plasma concentrations were found, then true tolerance would be demonstrated.

Enuresis. Because it provides the largest available body of data, the report of Rapoport et al. (42) on plasma tricyclic concentration of IMI and DMI in boys undergoing tricyclic treatment for enuresis will be reviewed in detail. After an initial single blind 2-week trial of placebo, children were placed on either IMI (75 mg hs) or DMI (75 mg hs) for 13 days while parents kept diaries of clinical response. Plasma for determination of drug concentration was obtained at 8:00 am on day 13. Both IMI and DMI were more effective than placebo but did not differ significantly from each other.

As seen in Figure 2, there was a wide range of plasma values, with a 15-fold difference between lowest and highest concentrations of DMI or of total DMI plus IMI. Plasma DMI also correlated significantly ($r = .59$; $n = 20$; $p < .01$) with continence on DMI medication. There was no evidence of a therapeutic window; that is, all children with 150 ng/ml or more of DMI or total (DMI plus IMI) showed some improvement. In the 40 IMI study patients, total (IMI plus DMI) correlated significantly with antienuretic effect ($r = .46$, $p < .01$), while plasma IMI and IMI/DMI ratio did not show significant association with clinical efficacy.

The relationship between clinical effect and plasma concentration of tricyclic treatment appears more complex, however, when follow-up data are considered. As shown in Figures 3, 4, and 5, when four of six "nonresponders" were brought up to higher plasma concentrations with increased maintenance doses, they continued to be incontinent. Four children (of 13) who were "transient" responders had increased plasma concentrations and were followed on the increased concentrations. A transient response was defined as greater than 50% dry nights for 2 weeks, with subsequent wearoff of effect. The group showed a transient response in spite of the maintenance of an increased plasma concentration. A small comparison group of good responders is also shown to indicate that there is no apparent alteration in plasma concentration in this group of subjects for whom IMI continued to be efficacious.

PLASMA CONCENTRATION AND ANTIDEPRESSANT EFFECT

Puig-Antich et al. report the antidepressant effect in relation to tricyclic plasma level in prepubertal children, although this is preliminary (37). In this report, 13 prepubertal children meeting the adult RDC for major depressive disorder were treated with a mean of 3.9 mg/kg/day of IMI (mean maintenance dose of 105 mg/day). In the first analysis, no significant correlation between change scores in the "Kiddie" SADS and plasma concentration (weeks 3, 4, and 5) was found, but a reanalysis, with an extreme value discarded, did show a significant relationship to clinical change. A nonparametric comparison of responders and nonresponders showed significant differences in plasma levels between the two groups ($p < .05$), with a cut-off of 146 ng/ml separating responders from nonresponders.

SUMMARY

The studies discussed in this chapter indicate there are both distinct clinical uses and pharmacologic effects of tricyclic antidepressants in children. In at least two disorders, enuresis and hyperkinetic behavior, the therapeutic effects of tricyclics appear to be immediate. This immediate action is in contrast to the delayed effects seen in the treatment of adult, and possibly childhood, depression. The mechanism of the antienuretic and antihyperkinetic effects might be related to the acute inhibitory action of tricyclics on monoamine neurotransmitter uptake. This can only be speculation, because available evidence of the pharmacologic and biochemical effects of tricyclics in these disorders is insufficient to identify a particular mechanism.

Side effects of tricyclics may also be different in children. The finding that children show an increase in supine and diastolic blood pressure following chronic tricyclic administration whereas adults show systolic hypotension needs explanation. The mechanism(s) of differing cardiovascular effects of tricyclics in adults and children is unknown and cannot, in any direct way, be associated with the monoamine uptake inhibitory actions of these drugs.

Recent pharmacokinetic studies of tricyclics have begun to provide information necessary to understand the mechanisms of these diverse drug actions. For instance, following a tertiary amine tricyclic, male children achieve relatively higher steady-state concentrations of the demethylated active metabolite than do adults. There is not, however, sufficient understanding of the relative effects of the different active forms to relate this pharmacokinetic difference to any differences in drug effects on cardiovascular function.

With respect to the relationship of steady-state concentration and drug effect, findings in children do not appear to be unique. However, adequate acute or single-dose studies of tricyclics in children are not available. Even with this limitation it appears unlikely that pharmacokinetic differences will provide an explanation for unique effects of tricyclics in children. Nonetheless, as part of any attempt to understand both the acute and chronic effects of these drugs, it is important to assess drug concentrations at the periods most relevant to clinical effect. This knowledge, combined with that of the pharmacodynamics of tricyclics in children (when such information becomes available), may be useful. This chapter reviewed studies that can help design future research. Thus, if one can achieve the same clinical effect using a tricyclic not subject to demethylation, it is likely that any differences observed between effects in children and adults can be attributed to pharmacodynamics (e.g., difference in drug-induced hormonal changes in pre- and postpubescent individuals).

The interesting finding of "wear-off" of the antienuretic effect of tricyclics in the presence of sustained plasma concentration of drug is evidence for pharmacodynamic change, since pharmacokinetic stability is demonstrated. Future studies need to define the different biochemical effects of acute and chronic treatment. Such differences may provide important clues to understanding the mode of action of tricyclics in enuresis and hyperactive behavior disorders.

Finally, it should be emphasized that the diagnostic, pharmacologic, and physiologic issues that have been discussed await confirmation and future study. Such work will require close collaboration between child psychiatrists, clinical pharmacologists, and basic scientists.

REFERENCES AND BIBLIOGRAPHY

1. Blackwell B, Currah J (1973): The psychopharmacology of nocturnal enuresis. In Kolvin I, MacKeith R, Meadow S, eds: Bladder Control and Enuresis (Clinics in Developmental Medicine No. 48/49) London, Heinemann.
2. Blumberg A, Klein D, Pollack M (1964): Effects of chlorimipramine and imipramine on

systolic blood pressure in psychiatric patients: Relationship to age, diagnosis and initial blood pressure. J Psychiatric Res 2:51–60.

3. Breger E (1962): Hydroxyzine hydrochloride and methylphenidate hydroxychloride in the management of enuresis. J Pediatr 61:443–447.

4. Conners C (1976): Classification and treatment of childhood depression and depressive equivalents. In Gallant D, Simpson G, eds: Depression: Behavioral, Biochemical, Diagnostic and Treatment Concepts. New York, Spectrum, pp 181–196.

5. DiMascio A, Soltys J (1970): Psychotropic drug side-effects in children. In DiMascio A, Shader P, eds: Psychotropic Drug Side-Effects: Clinical and Theoretical Perspectives. Baltimore, Williams & Wilkins.

6. Frommer E (1967): Treatment of childhood depression with antidepressant drugs. Br Med J 1:729–732.

7. General Practitioners Research Group (1970): Sedatives and stimulants compared in enuresis. Practitioner 204:584–590.

8. Gibaldi M, Levy G, McNamara P (1978): Effect of plasma protein and tissue binding on the biologic half life of drugs. Clin Pharmacol Ther 24:1–4.

9. Gillette J (1979): Biotransformation of drugs during aging. Fed Proc 38:1900–1909.

10. Gittelman-Klein R (1974): Pilot clinical trial of imipramine in hyperkinetic children. In Conners C, ed: Clinical Use of Stimulant Drugs in Children. The Hague, Excerpta Medica, pp 199–201.

11. Gittelman-Klein R, Klein D (1971): Controlled imipramine of school phobia. Arch Gen Psychiatry 25:204–207.

12. Glassman A, Bigger T, Giardina E, Kantor S, Perel J, Davies M (1979): The clinical characteristics of imipramine induced orthostatic hypotension. Lancet 1:468–472.

13. Glassman A, Perel J, Shostak M, Kantor S, Fleiss J (1977): Clinical implications of imipramine plasma levels for depressive illness. Arch Gen Psychiatry 34:197–204.

14. Graham P (1974): Depression in pre-pubertal children. Dev Med Child Neurol 16: 340–349.

15. Gram L, Sondergaard I, Christiansen J, Petersen G, Beck P, Reisby W, Ortmann J, Nagy A, Dencker S, Jacobsen O, Krautwald O (1977): Steady-state kinetics of imipramine in patients. Psychopharmacology 54:255–261.

16. Greenberg L, Yellin A (1975): Blood pressure and pulse changes in hyperactive children treated with imipramine and methylphenidate. Am J Psychiatry 132:1325–1326.

17. Greenberg L, Yellin A, Spring C, Metcalf M (1975): Clinical effects of imipramine and methylphenidate in hyperactive children. Int J Ment Health 4:144–156.

18. Gugler R, Shoeman D, Huffman D, Cohlmia J, Azarnoff D (1975): Pharmacokinetics of drugs in patients with the nephrotic syndrome. J Clin Invest 55:1182–1189.

19. Huessy H, Wright A (1970): The use of imipramine in children's behavior disorders. Acta Paedopsychiatrica 37:194–199.

20. Jandhyala B, Steenberg M, Perel J, Manian A, Buckley J (1977): Effects of several tricyclic antidepressants on the hemodynamics and myocardial contractility of anesthetized dogs. Eur J Pharmacol 42:403–410.

21. Koehl F, Wenzel J (1971): Severe postural hypotension due to imipramine therapy. Pediatrics 47:132–134.

22. Krakowski A (1965): Amitryptyline in treatment of hyperkinetic children. A double-blind study. Psychosomatics 6:355–360.

23. Kristiansen ES (1961): Cardiac complications during treatment with imipramine. Acta Psychiatry Scand 36:427–441.

24. Kuhn V, Kuhn R (1972): Drug therapy for depression in children: In Annel A, ed: Depressive States in Childhood and Adolescence. New York, Halsted Press.

25. Kupietz S, Balka E (1976): Alterations in vigilance performance of children receiving amitryptyline and methylphenidate pharmacotherapy. Psychopharmacology 50:24–33.

26. Lake R, Mikkelsen E, Rapoport J, Zavadil A, Kopin IJ (1980): The effect of imipramine on plasma NE and on blood pressure in enuretic boys. Clin Pharm Ther 26:647–653.

27. Ling W, Oftedal G, Weinberg W (1970): Depressive illness in childhood presenting as severe headache. Am J Dis Child 120:122–124.

28. McConaghy W (1969): A controlled trial of imipramine, amphetamine, pad and bell conditioning and random awakening in the treatment of nocturnal enuresis. Med J Austral 2:237–239.

29. McLean R (1960): Imipramine hydroxychloride (Tofranil) and enuresis. Am J Psychiatry 117:551.

30. Muscettola E, Goodwin F, Petter W, Claeys M, Markey S (1978): Imipramine and desimipramine in plasma and spinal fluid. Arch Gen Psychiatry 35:621–625.

31. Perel J, Irani F, Hurwic M, Glassman A, Manion A (1978): Tricyclic antidepressants: Relationships among pharmacokinetics, metabolism and clinical outcome. In Garratini S, ed: Depressive Disorders Symposium. New York, Schattauer-Verlag.

32. Piafsky K, Börgå O (1978): Plasma protein binding of basic drugs III: Importance of α_1-acid glycoprotein for interindividual variation. Clin Pharmacol Ther 22: 545–549.

33. Potter W, Calil H, Zavadil A, Jusko W, Sutfin T, Rapoport J, and Goodwin F (1980) Steady-state concentrations of hydroxylated metabolites of tricyclic antidepressants in patients: Relationship to clinical effect. Psychopharmacol Bull 16:32–34.

34. Potter WZ, Zovadil AP III, Kopin IJ Goodwin FK (1980): Single-dose kinetics predict steady-state concentrations of imipramine and desipramine. Arch Gen Psychiatry 37:314–320.

35. Poussaint A, Ditman D (1965): A controlled study of imipramine (Tofranil) in the treatment of childhood enuresis. J Pediatr 67:285–290.

36. Puig-Antich J, Balu S, Marx N, Greenhill L, Chambers W (1979): Prepubertal major depressive disorder: A pilot study. J Am Acad Child Psychiatry 17:695–797.

37. Puig-Antich J, Perel J, Lupatkin W, Chambers W, Shea C, Tabrizi M, Stiller R (1980): IMI and DMI plasma levels and clinical response in major depressive disorder in children. Psychopharmacol Bull 16: 25–26.

38. Quinn PO, Rapoport J (1975): A one year follow-up of hyperactive boys treated with imipramine or methylphenidate. Am J Psychiatry 132:241–245.

39. Rapoport J (1965): Childhood behavior and learning problems treated with imipramine. Int J Neuropsychiatry 1:635–642.

40. Rapoport J (1976): Pediatric psychopharmacology and childhood depression. In Klein D, Gittelman-Klein R, eds: Progress in Psychiatric Drug Treatment, New York, Brunner-Mazel.

41. Rapoport J, Quinn P, Bradbard G, Riddle K, Brooks E (1974): Imipramine and methylphenidate treatment of hyperactive boys. Arch Gen Psychiatry 30:789–794.

42. Rapoport J, Mikkelsen E, Zavadil A, Nee L, Gruneu C, Mendelsen W, Gillin JC (1980): Enuresis II: Psychopathology, plasma tricyclic concentration and antienuretic responses. Arch Gen Psychiatry 37: 1146–1152.

43. Saraf K, Klein D, Gittelman-Klein R, Groff S (1974): Imipramine side-effects in children. Psychopharmacology 37:265–274.

44. Saraf K, Klein D, Gittelman-Klein R, Goodwin W, Greenhill P (1978): EKG effects of imipramine treatment in children. J Am Acad Child Psychiatry 17:60–70.

45. Spitzer R, Endicott J, Robins E (1975): Research diagnostic criteria (RDC). Psychopharmacol Bull 3:22–25.

46. Stephenson J (1979): Physiological and pharmacological basis for the chemotherapy of enuresis. Psychol Med 9:1–5.

47. Waizer J, Hofman S, Polizos P, Engelhardt D (1974): Outpatient treatment of hyperactive school children with imipramine. Am J Psychiatry 131:587–591.

48. Weinberg W, Rutman J, Sullivan L, et al. (1973): Depression in children referred to an education diagnostic center: Diagnosis and treatment. J Pediatr 83:1065–1072.

49. Werry J, Dowrick P, Lampen E, Vamus M (1975): Imipramine in enuresis: Psychological and physiological effects. J Child Psychol Psychiatry 16:289–299.

50. Winsberg B, Bialer I, Klutch A, Perel J (1973): Imipramine fate and behavior in hyperactive children. Psychopharmacol Bull 9:45–46.

51. Winsberg B, Perel J, Hurwiz M, Klutch A (1974): Imipramine protein binding and pharmacokinetics in children. In Forrest I, Usdin E, eds: The Phenothiazines and Structurally Related Drugs. New York, Raven Press.

52. Winsberg B, Bialer I, Kupietz S, Tobias J (1972): Effects of imipramine and dextro-amphetamine on behavior of neuropsychiatrically impaired children. Am J Psychiatry 128:1425–1432.

53. Winsberg B, Goldstein S, Yepes L, Perel J (1975): Imipramine and electrocardiographic abnormalities in hyperactive children. Am J Psychiatry 132:542–545.

54. Yepes L, Balka E, Winsberg B, Bialer I (1977): Amitryptyline and methylphenidate treatment of behaviorally disordered children. J Child Psychol Psychiatry 18:39–52.

9

EFFECTS OF AGE
ON THE PHARMACOLOGY
OF TRICYCLIC ANTIDEPRESSANTS

Robert O. Friedel

This chapter will focus on the pertinent variables affecting pharmacologic response to tricyclic antidepressants in elderly depressed patients. The incidence of severe depression appears to increase with aging (24), and the relative frequency of presumptive biologic subtypes of depression also appear to change with the aging process (31). Also, there appear to be certain age-related biochemical changes occurring in the central nervous system (CNS) that may have a direct bearing on the biologic bases of depressive subtypes in elderly patients. Possibly the most important of these changes are the decreased synthesis and hydrolysis of acetylcholine observed in old animals, associated with increased sensitivity of cholinergic receptors to both agonists and antagonists (8), and the increase in monoamine oxidase levels observed in elderly patients associated with a decreased CNS norepinephrine concentration (28). Finally, there are data suggesting that some pharmacokinetic processes appear to change significantly with age (7, 9, 26, 29).

From these data, one can derive three hypotheses. First, some subtypes of depression in the elderly may have different biochemical bases than in younger depressed patients, and, consequently, the response to tricyclic antidepressants may be altered in patients with these different depressive subtypes. Second, with age-related changes in the structure and chemistry of the CNS, the pharmacodynamic response of depressions of the same subtypes to antidepressants may be different in young and old patients.

From the Department of Psychiatry, Medical College of Virginia, Virginia Commonwealth University, Richmond, Virginia.

Third, in patients with depressions of the same biologic subtype, and the same pharmacodynamic response to similar levels of tricyclic antidepressants, pharmacokinetic changes in the elderly subjects may result in alterations in plasma and CNS drug and metabolite levels that result in altered therapeutic and toxic responses. The remainder of this chapter reviews available evidence relevant to these three hypotheses.

AGE-RELATED DIFFERENCES IN BIOLOGIC SUBTYPES OF DEPRESSION

The contention that some elderly patients suffer from different biologic types of depressions than do younger patients has not been tested directly. However, if one assumes that the effects of tricyclic antidepressants on depresssion is related to their specific actions on different neurotransmitter pathways in the central nervous system, a careful comparison of the response of elderly and younger subjects to tricyclic antidepressants may provide information related to this hypothesis. A careful review of the literature revealed 16 controlled studies that evaluated the effects of tricyclic antidepressants in elderly depressed patients. Eight of these studies involved tricyclic–placebo comparisons (1, 6, 14, 18, 20, 25, 27, 33), and in an additional eight studies a tricyclic antidepressant was compared to another tricyclic or to some other psychoactive agent (3, 5, 13, 15–17, 19, 32). Data on the efficacy and relative efficacy of tricyclic antidepressants from these studies are compared to similar data compiled on nonelderly subject populations (22) in Tables 1 and 2.

These comparisons must be viewed with caution because of the relative paucity of studies involving elderly subjects and because in no studies reported were diagnostic CNS changes and pharmacokinetic variables controled.

TABLE 1. Controlled Studies Comparing Tricyclics with Placebo in Elderly and Nonelderly Subjects

	Nonelderly[a]		Elderly[b]	
Drug studied	Superior to placebo	Not superior	Superior to placebo	Not superior
Imipramine	30	20	3	1
Amitriptyline	14	6	1	0
Nortriptyline	5	3	1	1
Amitriptyline and perphenazine	4	1	1	0
Totals	53	30	6	2

[a]Data adapted from Morris and Beck (22).
[b]Data summarized from eight controlled studies (1, 6, 14, 18, 20, 25, 26, 33).

TABLE 2. Controlled Studies Comparing Tricylics with Other Psychoactive Agents in Elderly and Nonelderly Subjects

Drugs compared	Nonelderly[a]			Elderly[b]		
	Superior	No difference	Inferior	Superior	No difference	Inferior
Amitriptyline vs imipramine	5	4	2	2	0	0
Amitriptyline vs doxepin	1	4	3	0	1	0
Amitriptyline vs amitriptyline and chlordiazepoxide	0	0	0	0	0	1
Desipramine vs nortriptyline	0	0	0	0	1	0
Amitriptyline and perphenazine vs chlordiazepoxide	0	0	0	1	0	0
Protriptyline vs nortriptyline and fluphenazine	0	0	0	0	1	0
Protriptyline vs thiothixene	0	0	0	0	1	0

[a]Data adapted from Morris and Beck (22).
[b]Data summarized from eight controlled studies (3, 5, 13, 15–17, 19, 32).

Although the overall summarization of these data did not indicate any significant age-related differences in the efficacy or relative efficacy of tricyclic antidepressants, several individual studies have produced results that did suggest such differences. Chesrow et al. (6) compared nortriptyline with placebo in depressed subjects of all ages and found nortriptyline to be less effective in subjects over 65 years of age. Kiloh et al. (20) compared imipramine with placebo and found that patients over age 40 years responded better than younger patients. In support of these earlier findings, the NIMH Collaborative Depression Study Group (25), which compared imipramine, chlorpromazine, and placebo, found that imipramine was an effective antidepressant in patients over age 40 years but not in younger patients. However, Wittenborn et al. (32) compared imipramine, amitriptyline, and thioridazine and found older patients responded poorly to imipramine. In a comparison of amitriptyline, trimipramine, and placebo in depressed patients, Rickels et al. (27) found no difference in response in patients both younger and older than 40 years of age.

In summary, studies comparing the efficacy and relative efficacy of tricyclic antidepressants in elderly and younger subjects have not revealed any consistent age-related differences in clinical response. However, studies involving elderly subjects are few in number, poorly controlled, and some individual studies suggest that such age-related differences may indeed occur. If this is the case, such studies may provide an indirect approach to evaluating the question of age-related differences in the biologic bases of depressive subtypes.

EFFECTS OF AGE-RELATED CNS BIOCHEMICAL CHANGES ON THE PHARMACODYNAMIC RESPONSE OF DEPRESSED ELDERLY PATIENTS TO TRICYCLIC ANTIDEPRESSANTS

Although there is increasing interest in developmental psychopharmacology, much of the work has been directed at the early end of the developmental life cycle (21, 30). Consequently, there are few data from either human or animal studies relevant to the question of alterations in pharmacodynamic response to tricyclic antidepressants in elderly populations. There is evidence suggesting an increased tendency for elderly patients to develop anticholinergic toxicity secondary to the administration of tricyclic antidepressants (11), but this does not speak to the issue of age-related variation in therapeutic response to these substances. Nonetheless, given the changes noted above in cholinergic, noradrenergic, and possibly other CNS neurotransmitter levels and in receptor sensitivity in aged humans and animals, it is most likely that many pharmacodynamic responses to tricyclic antidepressants do change significantly with age.

EFFECTS OF AGE-RELATED PHARMACOKINETIC CHANGES ON THE RESPONSE OF DEPRESSED ELDERLY PATIENTS TO TRICYCLIC ANTIDEPRESSANTS

Recent reviews have documented clearly the fact that there are substantial alterations in the absorption, distribution, metabolism, and excretion of drugs in elderly patients (7, 9, 26, 29). Although no generalization can be derived from these data regarding age-related changes in drug absorption, there does appear to be a consistent trend toward increased distribution volumes of lipid soluble drugs and decreased distribution of polar drugs as patients age. There also are data suggesting that the metabolism and excretion of many drugs is decreased in some elderly subjects. In conclusion, it is difficult to predict what the sum of these changes will be on plasma and tissue levels of drugs and their metabolites in elderly subjects; each drug must be evaluated separately. Nonetheless, it is safe to assume that in many elderly patients significant pharmacokinetic effects do occur with resultant alterations in drug response.

Fortunately, there are some data available on the effects of aging on the pharmacokinetics of tricyclic antidepressants. Nies et al. (23) have reported that elderly patients treated with fixed doses of imipramine or amitriptyline developed higher steady-state plasma levels of imipramine, desipramine, and amitriptyline than younger patients. Elderly patients treated with amitriptyline did not achieve steady-state plasma levels of nortriptyline any higher than young patients, suggesting that the metabolism of nortriptyline is less affected in elderly subjects than that of desipramine, the other monomethylated tricyclic studied. In addition, the mean half-lives of imipramine and amitriptyline and the apparent half-life of desipramine were found to be increased significantly in the elderly group, but the apparent half-life of nortriptyline was not. Friedel et al. (12) have recently reported significant positive correlations of age with desipramine plasma levels after 2 and 3 weeks of treatment. This provides further evidence that desipramine metabolism becomes impaired in some patients as age increases.

Åsberg et al. (2) have reported findings consistent with those of Nies et al. (23) that nortriptyline metabolism is unaffected by age. In addition, Braithwaite et al. (4) have recently reported a significant correlation of amitriptyline steady-state plasma levels with age, but no significant correlation between nortriptyline steady-state plasma levels and age in patients receiving amitriptyline or nortriptyline. These findings are consistent with those of Nies et al. (23). However, Braithwaite et al. (4) did find significant increases in the variability of steady-state plasma levels of amitriptyline and nortriptyline in depressed patients over 55 years of age treated with each of these drugs. Combining the results of five single-dose nortriptyline studies, these authors also found a significant positive correlation between plasma nortriptyline half-life and age but no such correlation between plasma nortriptyline clearance and age.

These data are hardly conclusive regarding the effects of aging on the pharmacokinetics of tricyclic antidepressants. However, it appears that steady-state plasma levels of amitriptyline, imipramine, and desipramine may increase with age, whereas that of nortriptyline seems more stable. There also is more variability in tricyclic antidepressant steady-state plasma levels, half-life, and clearance in elderly than in younger patients. Monitoring tricyclic steady-state plasma levels in elderly depressed patients may therefore increase therapeutic response and decrease toxicity. This is supported by the findings of Friedel and Raskind (10), who studied 15 elderly depressed patients treated with doxepin and found significantly higher plasma levels of doxepin and desmethyldoxepin in those patients who had a favorable clinical response than in those who did not. A marked disparity between doxepin dosage and steady-state plasma levels in a number of subjects also suggested considerable interpatient variability in pharmacokinetic processes in these patients, a finding in agreement with those cited previously.

CONCLUSION

This review indicates clearly there are few data available regarding the effects of age on the pharmacology of tricyclic antidepressants. The contention that some elderly patients suffer from depressive subtypes that are biologically different than those found in younger patients is presently conjectured. Some pharmacodynamic and pharmacokinetic responses of tricyclic antidepressants may be altered in elderly patients.

REFERENCES AND BIBLIOGRAPHY

1. Abraham HC, Kanter VB, Rosen I, et al. (1963): A controlled clinical trial of imipramine (Tofranil) with outpatients. Br J Psychiatry 109:286–293.
2. Åsberg M, Cronholm B, Sjöqvist F, Tuck O (1971): Relationship between plasma level and therapeutic effect of nortriptyline. Br Med J 3:331–334.
3. Beber CR (1971): Treating anxiety and depression in the elderly: a double-blind crossover evaluation of two widely used tranquilizers. J Florida AM 58:35–38.
4. Braithwaite R, Montgomery S, Dawling S: Age, depression and tricyclic antidepressants. Presented at symposium, Drugs in the Elderly, Dundee, Scotland, 1977.
5. Brodie NH, McGhie RL, O'Hara H, Valle-Jones JC, Schiff AA (1975): Anxiety depression in elderly patients: A double-blind comparative study of fluphenazine, nortriptyline and promazine. Practitioner 215:660–664.
6. Chesrow EI, Kaplitz SE, Breme JT, Sabatini R, Vetra H, Marquardt GH (1964): Nortriptyline for the treatment of anxiety and depression in chronically ill and geriatric patients. J Am Geriatr Soc 12:271–277.
7. Crooks J, O'Malley K, Sevenson IH (1976): Pharmacokinetics in the elderly. Clin Pharmacokinet 1:280–296.
8. Domino EE, Dren AT, Giardina WJ (1978): Biochemical and neurotransmitter changes in the aging brain. In Lipton MA, DiMascio A, Killam KF, eds: Psychopharmacology: A Generation of Progress. New York, Raven Press.
9. Friedel RO (1978): Pharmacokinetics in the geropsychiatric patient. In Lipton MA, DiMascio A, Killam KF, eds.: Psychopharmacology: A Generation of Progress, New York, Raven Press.
10. Friedel RO, Raskind MA (1975): Relationship of blood levels of Sinequan to clinical effects in the treatment of depression in aged patients. In Mendels J, ed: Sinequan: A Monograph of Recent Clinical Studies, Princeton, New Jersey, Excerpta Medica.
11. Friedel RO, Raskind MA (1977): Psychopharmacology of Aging. In Elias MF, Eleftherion BE, Elias DK, eds: Special Review of Experimental Aging Research: Progress in Biology, Bar Harbor, E.A.R.
12. Friedel RO, Veith RC, Bloom B, Bielski RJ (1979): Desipramine plasma levels and clinical response in depressed outpatients. Commun Psychopharmacol 3:81–87.
13. Grof P, Saxena B, Cantor R, Daigle L, Hetherington D, Haines T (1974): Doxepin versus amitriptyline in depression: A sequential double-blind study. Curr Ther Res 16:470–476.
14. Haider I (1967): Amitriptyline and perphenazine in depressive illness: a controlled trial. Br J Psychiatry 113:195–199.
15. Haider I (1967): Combination of amitriptyline and chlordiazepoxide in depressive states. Br J Clin Pract 21:39–40.
16. Haider I (1968): A comparative investigation of desipramine and nortriptyline in the treatment of depression. Br J Psychiatry 114:1293–1294.

17. Hordern A, Burt CG, Holt NE (1965): Depressive States: A Pharmacotherapeutic Study. Springfield, Illinois, Charles C. Thomas.

18. Kernohan WJ, Chambers JL, Wilson WT, Daugherty JF (1967): Effects of nortriptyline on the mental and social adjustment of geriatric patients in a mental hospital. J Am Geriatr Soc 15:196–202.

19. Kiev A (1972): Double-blind comparison of thiothixene and protriptyline in psychotic depression. Dis Nerv Syst 33:811–816.

20. Kiloh LG, Ball JRP, Garside RF (1962): Prognostic factors in treatment of depressive states with imipramine. Br Med J 1:1225–1227.

21. Mabry PD, Campbell BA (1977): Developmental Psychopharmacology. In Iversen LL, Iversen SD, Snyder SH, eds: Handbook of Psychopharmacology, Vol. 7, Principles of Behavioral Pharmacology, Plenum Press, NY.

22. Morris JB, Beck, AT (1974): The efficacy of antidepressant drugs: A review of research (1958 to 1972). Arch Gen Psychiatry 30:667–674.

23. Nies A, Robinson DS, Friedman MI, Green R, Cooper TB, Ravaris CL, Ives JO (1977): Relationship between age and tricyclic antidepressant plasma levels. Am J Psychiatry 134:790–793.

24. Post F (1976): Diagnosis of depression in geriatric patients and treatment modalities appropriate for the population. In Gallant DM, Simpson CM, eds.: Depression: Behavioral, Biochemical, Diagnostic and Treatment Concepts, New York, Spectrum Publications.

25. Raskin A, Schulterbrandt JC, Reatig N, Chase C, McKeon JJ (1970): Differential response to chlorpromazine, imipramine and placebo. Arch Gen Psychiatry 23:164–174.

26. Richey FP, Bender AD (1977): Pharmacokinetic consequences of aging. Ann Rev Pharmacol Toxicol 17:49–65.

27. Rickels K, Gordon PE, Weise CC, et al. (1970): Amitriptyline and trimipramine in neurotic depressed outpatients: A collaborative study. Am J Psychiatry 127:208–218.

28. Robinson DS (1975): Changes in monoamine oxidase and monoamines with human development and aging. Fed Proc 34:103–107.

29. Triggs EJ, Nation RL, Long A, Ashley JJ (1975): Pharmacokinetics in the elderly. J Clin Pharmacol 8:55–62.

30. Werboff J (1978): Developmental psychopharmacology. In Clark WG, Del Guidice J, eds: Principles of Psychopharmacology, 2nd ed. New York, Academic Press.

31. Winokur G, Behar D, Vanvalkenburg C, Lowry M (1978): Is a familiar definition of depression both feasible and valid? J Nerv Ment Dis 166:764–768.

32. Wittenborn JR, Kiremite N, Weber E (1973): The choice of alternative antidepressants. J Nerv Ment Dis 156:97–108.

33. Zung WWK, Giaturco D, Pfeiffer E, Wang HS, Whanger A, Bridge TP, Potkin SG (1976): Pharmacology of depression in the aged: Evaluation of Gerovital H3 as an antidepressant drug. Psychosomatics 15:127–131.

10

TRICYCLIC ANTIDEPRESSANTS AND THE AGING PROCESS: DISCUSSION OF SELECTED PHARMACODYNAMIC AND PHARMACOKINETIC ISSUES

Joseph J. Schildkraut

This chapter addresses four rather fundamental issues, and aspects of our research on tricyclic antidepressant drugs will serve as illustrative material. The first point to be made is a rather trivial one but one that deserves to be repeated in this context, namely, that tricyclic antidepressant drugs have differences as well as similarities in their pharmacodynamic effects and that the tricyclic antidepressants produce many other pharmacologic effects in addition to inhibiting the uptake of one or another of the monoamines.

The second set of comments will be with respect to the differences observed in the effects of tricyclic antidepressants after acute administration when compared to the effects observed after chronic administration. Points will be illustrated principally by referring to the effects of these drugs on the noradrenergic neuronal system, but by no means is this the only neuronal system on which these drugs act.

The third issue is the role of the biochemical and physiologic status of the patient in determining the clinical effects of these drugs. Here reference will be made to data on the use of pretreatment measures of urinary 3-methoxy-4-hydroxyphenylglycol (MHPG) as a predictor of differential responses to treatment with one or another tricyclic or tetracyclic antidepressant drug.

In the final section consideration is given to the important effects of aging on the metabolism of tricyclic antidepressants, by presenting a case

From the Harvard Medical School and the Neuropsychopharmacology Laboratory, Massachusetts Mental Health Center, Boston, Massachusetts.

This work was supported in part by grant MH15413 from the National Institute of Mental Health.

study of a 68-year-old woman that illustrates the possible effects of aging on the pharmacokinetics of tricyclic antidepressant drugs and further documents the clinical importance of measuring plasma tricyclic antidepressant blood levels, particularly in elderly patients.

DIFFERENCES IN THE EFFECTS OF ACUTELY ADMINISTERED TRICYCLIC ANTIDEPRESSANT DRUGS ON THE UPTAKE AND METABOLISM OF NOREPINEPHRINE IN RAT BRAIN

The effects of tricyclic antidepressants administered acutely on norepinephrine uptake and metabolism in brain in vitro and in vivo have been examined by many investigators (23). These studies have demonstrated an inhibition of norepinephrine uptake and an alteration in its pathways of metabolism after administration of one or another tricyclic antidepressant drug.

In studies performed in our laboratory a number of years ago, we examined the uptake and metabolism of intracisternally administered tritiated norepinephrine in rat brain after acute administration of a number of clinically effective tricyclic antidepressant drugs (27). As described in Table 1, tricyclic antidepressant drugs were administered by intraperitoneal injection 90 minutes before the intracisternal injection of tritiated norepinephrine, and animals were killed 6 minutes after the intracisternal injection to determine the effects of the drugs on the initial uptake and metabolism of tritiated norepinephrine. As shown in Table 1,

TABLE 1. Effects of Tricyclic Antidepressants on the Uptake and Metabolism of NE-^{3}H in Rat Brain

Drug	NE-^{3}H	NMN-^{3}H	DCM-^{3}H	Total DOM-^{3}H	Free DOM-^{3}H
Desmethylimipramine	71 ± 2^a	196 ± 7^a	52 ± 2^a	102 ± 3	100 ± 6
Protriptyline	67 ± 5^a	174 ± 11^a	45 ± 4^a	92 ± 5	98 ± 5
Imipramine	81 ± 5^b	176 ± 8^a	50 ± 3^a	94 ± 7	100 ± 12
Nortriptyline	80 ± 3^a	151 ± 6^a	48 ± 2^a	93 ± 3	102 ± 9
Amitriptyline	100 ± 2	123 ± 4^a	74 ± 3^a	95 ± 2	94 ± 5

Drugs were administered as hydrochloride salts (25 mg/kg) 90 minutes before intracisternal injection of norepinephrine-^{3}H, and animals were killed 6 minutes after the intracisterinal injection. Norepinephine-^{3}H and metabolite concentrations were measured in whole rat brain by methods cited in reference listed below. Data are expressed as a percentage of matched control means $\pm$ standard errors of the means. Abbreviation: NE-^{3}H, tritiated norepinephrine; NMN-^{3}H, tritiated normetanephrine; DCM-^{3}H, tritiated deaminated catechol metabolites, i.e., 3,4-dihydroxymandelic acid and 3,4-dihydroxyphenylglycol; total DOM-^{3}H, total tritiated deaminated O-methylated metabolites, i.e., 3-methoxy-4-hydroxymandelic acid (VMA), 3-methoxy-4-hydroxyphenylglycol (MHPG), and the sulfate conjugate of MHPG; free DOM-^{3}H, tritiated VMA and unconjugated MHPG. (Data reproduced from Schildkraut, Dodge, Logue [1969]: J Psychiat Res 7:29–34.)

$^a p < .001$ when compared with matched control mean values.

$^b p < .01$ when compared with matched control mean values.

desmethylimipramine, imipramine, protriptyline, and nortriptyline all inhibited the uptake of norepinephrine in brain as evidenced by the decrease in levels of tritiated norepinephrine when compared with control values. A greater decrease was observed with desmethylimipramine and protriptyline than with imipramine and nortriptyline, but all of these compounds caused statistically significant changes. In contrast, prior treatment with amitriptyline did not inhibit norepinephrine uptake. Whereas amitriptyline has been reported to inhibit the uptake of norepinephrine in brain under some conditions, and amitriptyline can be metabolized to nortriptyline that inhibits the uptake of norepinephrine in our experiments, our data indicate that under the conditions of this experiment amitriptyline differs from certain other tricyclic antidepressants with respect to its effects on norepinephrine uptake in the brain.

All of the tricyclic antidepressants we studied, including amitriptyline, cause statistically significant decreases in levels of tritiated deaminated catechol metabolites and increases in the levels of tritiated normetanephrine in the brain. Desmethylimipramine, imipramine, protriptyline, and nortriptyline all appear to cause comparable decreases in levels of tritiated deaminated catechol metabolites in brain. The changes in metabolism of tritiated norepinephrine (i.e., the decrease in tritiated deaminated catechol metabolites and the increase in tritiated normetanephrine) caused by amitriptyline also reached high levels of statistical significance ($p < .001$), but were smaller than the changes produced by the other drugs studied under comparable conditions (see Table 1).

DIFFERENCES IN THE EFFECTS OF ACUTE VERSUS CHRONIC ADMINISTRATION OF TRICYCLIC ANTIDEPRESSANT DRUGS ON NOREPINEPHRINE TURNOVER IN BRAIN

In our studies comparing the effects of acute and chronic administration of tricyclic antidepressant drugs (18, 30, 31), we found that the inhibition of norepinephrine uptake in brain and the changes in its metabolism were qualitatively similar after acute or chronic administration of imipramine and several other tricyclic antidepressants, although in some instances more pronounced effects were observed after chronic treatment. However, in these as well as in subsequent studies, we did observe differences in the effects of acute and chronic administration of tricyclic antidepressants on norepinephrine turnover. The following is a brief summary of this research.

Acute administration of imipramine or desmethylimipramine slows the disappearance of intracisternally administered norepinephrine-^{3}H from rat brain (Figure 1), suggesting a decrease in turnover of norepinephrine (7, 29). This decrease in turnover could reflect a decrease in the rate of discharge of norepinephrine from presynaptic noradrenergic neurons,

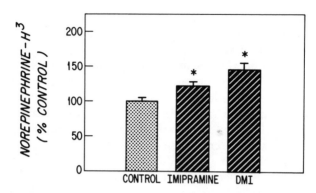

FIGURE 1. Disappearance of NE-^{3}H from rat brain after acute imipramine and DMI. Imipramine hydrochloride (25 mg/kg), desmethylimipramine hydrochloride (25 mg/kg), or isotonic saline (control) was administered by intraperitoneal injection 90 minutes after the intracisternal injection of norepinephrine-^{3}H, and animals were sacrificed 270 minutes after the intracisternal injection. Results represent the means of at least five determinations and are expressed as percentages of the control mean (100%) ± standard errors of the means; *$p < .01$ when compared with control values. (Data reproduced from Schildkraut, Schanberg, Breese, Kopin [1967]: Am J Psychiat 124:600–608.)

possibly as a result of presynaptic or postsynaptic feedback inhibition (26). Since reuptake into the presynaptic neuron is thought to be the major process for terminating the physiologic activity of extraneuronal norepinephrine, the inhibition of uptake produced by these drugs may increase concentration of norepinephrine at receptors and, thus, by a feedback mechanism decrease the rate of norepinephrine discharge from the presynaptic neuron. Such feedback inhibition would attenuate the increase in noradrenergic activity resulting from the inhibition of norepinephrine uptake produced by acute administration of these drugs, and this might help to explain why clinical antidepressant effects are not observed after acute administration of these tricyclic antidepressants. Approximately 10 years ago, we therefore began to explore the possible differences between the effects of acute and chronic administration of imipramine on the turnover of norepinephrine in rat brain (30, 31).

In one series of experiments, imipramine (10 mg/kg) or isotonic saline was administered by intraperitoneal injection to three groups of rats: one group was treated with a single dose; another group was treated twice daily for 10 days; and a third group was treated twice daily for 3 weeks. Six hours after the last intraperitoneal injection, tritiated norepinephrine was administered by intracisternal injection, and one group of animals was killed 6 minutes after the intracisternal injection to examine the effects of imipramine on the initial uptake of norepinephrine-^{3}H, another group 270 minutes after the intracisternal injection to examine the effects of the drug on the subsequent disappearance of norepinephrine-³H in rat brains. As shown in Figure 2, a single dose of imipramine inhibited the uptake of norepinephrine in brain as reflected by the lower concentrations of norepinephrine-³H in the brains of animals killed 6 minutes after the intracisternal injection. However, animals treated with a single dose of imipramine and killed 270 minutes after the administration of norepinephrine-³H had higher levels of norepinephrine-³H in the brain than did the controls. Acute administration of imipramine thus appeared to slow the rate of disappearance of norepinephrine-³H from the brain, since animals treated with a single dose of imipramine had lower levels of norepinephrine-³H in the brain than did controls at the earlier time and higher levels of norepinephrine-³H than did controls at the later time.

After 3 weeks of treatment with imipramine the uptake of norepinephrine-³H in brain remained inhibited, as evidenced by the lower levels of norepinephrine-³H in the brains of animals treated with imipramine and killed 6 minutes after the intracisternal injection. However,

FIGURE 2. Uptake (hatched shading) and disappearance (dotted shading) of NE-³H from rat brain after acute and chronic imipramine. In a series of experiments, imipramine hydrochloride (10 mg/kg) was administered by intraperitoneal injection to three groups of animals: one group was treated with a single dose; another group was treated twice daily for 10 days; and third group was treated twice daily for 3 weeks. Controls received isotonic saline according to the same schedule. In all experiments norepinephrine-³H was administered by intracisternal injection 6 hours after the last drug injection, and animals were sacrificed 6 or 270 minutes after administration of norepinephrine-³H. Results represent the means of 13 to 20 determinations and are expressed as percentages of the control means (100%) ± standard errors of the means. *$p < .05$ when compared to control values; **$p < .01$ when compared to control values. (Data reproduced from Schildkraut, Winokur, Applegate [1970]: Science 168:867–869; and Schildkraut, Winokur, Draskoczy, Hensle [1971]: Am J Psychiat 27:1032–1039.)

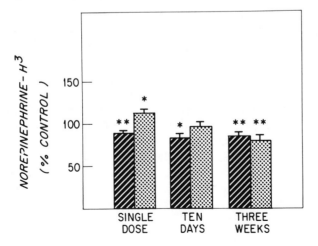

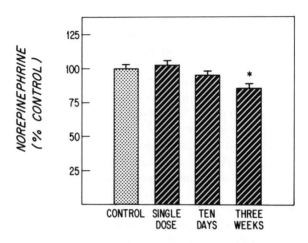

FIGURE 3. Endogenous norepinephrine in rat brain after acute and chronic imipramine. These experiments are described in the text and in Figure 2. Results are expressed as percentages of the control means (100%) ± standard errors of the means. *$p < .01$ when compared to control values. (Data reproduced from Schildkraut, Winokur, Draskoczy, Hensle [1971]: Am J Psychiat 127:1032–1039.)

residual levels of norepinephrine-^{3}H in brain (relative to control values) were even lower in animals given long-term treatment with imipramine and killed 270 minutes after the intracisternal injection, indicating that the rate of disappearance of norepinephrine-^{3}H from the brain was no longer slowed and possibly even accelerated (Figure 2). After 10 days of treatment with imipramine, the rate of disappearance of norepinephrine-^{3}H from brain was slower than after 3 weeks of treatment but faster than after a single dose (Figure 2), indicating that the change in the rate of disappearance of norepinephrine-^{3}H from rat brain develops gradually during chronic administration of imipramine.

As shown in Figure 3, the level of endogenous norepinephrine in rat brain was not altered by a single intraperitoneal injection of imipramine (10 mg/kg) but was significantly reduced after 3 weeks of treatment (10 mg/kg twice daily). Intermediate levels of norepinephrine were observed in brains of animals treated with imipramine for 10 days. This decrease in endogenous norepinephrine in rat brain after chronic administration of imipramine could reflect an enhanced rate of norepinephrine use in relation to its rate of synthesis.

In more recent studies (19), we have compared the effects of acute and chronic administration of imipramine and other tricyclic antidepressants on the levels of 3-methoxy-4-hydroxyphenylglycol sulfate (MHPG-SO$_4$) in rat brain. Since MHPG-SO$_4$ has been shown to be the major metabolite of norepinephrine in rat brain (21), measures of MHPG-SO$_4$ may provide an index of norepinephrine turnover in the brain (13).

TABLE 2. The Effects of Acute Administration of Tricyclic Antidepressants on the Levels of MHPG-SO$_4$ in Rat Brain

	Experiment 1		Experiment 2	
	MHPG-SO$_4$		MHPG-SO$_4$	
Drug	(pmol/g brain)	(Percent of control)	(pmol/g brain)	(Percent of control)
Saline	480 ± 13	100 ± 2.7	442 ± 14	100 ± 3.2
Desmethylimipramine	384 ± 19^a	80 ± 4.0^a	374 ± 16^b	85 ± 3.6^b
Imipramine	415 ± 16^b	86 ± 3.3^b	372 ± 18^b	84 ± 4.0^b
Nortriptyline	441 ± 18	92 ± 3.8	382 ± 27	86 ± 6.1
Amitriptyline	487 ± 15	101 ± 3.1	425 ± 27	96 ± 6.1

Desmethylimipramine hydrochloride (10 mg/kg), imipramine hydrochloride (10 mg/kg) nortriptyline hydrochloride (10 mg/kg), or amitriptyline hydrochloride (10 mg/kg) were administered by intraperitoneal injection. Control animals received saline (2ml/kg). Animals were killed 4 hours after drug injections in experiment 1, and 6 hours after drug injections in experiment 2. Each group contained 8 to 14 animals. Results are expressed as mean ± standard error of the means. (Data reproduced from Roffman, Kling, Cassens, Orsulak, Reigle, Schildkraut [1977]: Comm Psychopharmacol 1:195–206.)

^{a}p < .001 compared to control values.

^{b}p < .01 compared to control values.

Data presented in Table 2 show that the levels of MHPG-SO$_4$ in rat brain are significantly decreased after acute administration of desmethylimipramine (10 mg/kg) or imipramine (10 mg/kg) and tend to be decreased after nortriptyline (10 mg/kg), but not after amitriptyline (10 mg/kg). In animals killed 4 hours after drug administration (experiment 1) the most pronounced effects are produced by desmethylimipramine; but 6 hours after drug administration (experiment 2), desmethylimipramine and imipramine produce similar decreases in MHPG-SO$_4$, while nortriptyline also tends to decrease MHPG-SO$_4$. Amitriptyline has no meaningful effect on MHPG-SO$_4$ levels either 4 or 6 hours after acute administration (Table 2).

In contrast, as shown in Table 3, when these tricyclic antidepressants are administered chronically, significant increases in levels of MHPG-SO$_4$ are observed with desmethylimipramine and imipramine. Under these conditions, levels of MHPG-SO$_4$ are slightly, but not significantly, increased after nortriptyline and amitriptyline (Table 3).

These results are consistent with previous findings indicating that acutely administered desmethylimipramine or imipramine, but not amitriptyline, decreased the formation of radioactively labeled norepinephrine and its major metabolites (including MHPG) from radioactively labeled precursors (14, 15). These findings may be related to our earlier observations (Table 1) demonstrating that, under similar conditions, the uptake of intracisternally administered norepinephrine-^{3}H was inhibited by desmethylimipramine or imipramine, but not by amitriptyline (Table 1).

TABLE 3. THe Effects of Chronic Administration of Tricyclic Antidepressants on the Levels of MHPG-SO$_4$ in Rat Brain

Drug	MHPG-SO$_4$	
	(pmol/g brain)	(% of control)
Saline	455 ± 15	100 ± 3.3
Desmethylimipramine	538 ± 18^a	118 ± 4.0^a
Imipramine	542 ± 26^b	119 ± 5.7^b
Nortriptyline	493 ± 21	108 ± 4.6
Amitriptyline	507 ± 15	111 ± 3.3

Desmethylimipramine hydrochloride (10 mg/kg), imipramine hydrochloride (10 mg/kg), nortriptyline hydrochloride (10 mg/kg), or amitriptyline hydrochloride (10 mg/kg) were administered twice daily for 2 weeks. Control animals received saline (2 ml/kg) according to the same schedule as the drug treated groups. Animals were killed on the 15th day of treatment 6 hours after the 29th injection. Each group contained 12 to 14 animals. Results are expressed as means ± standard errors of the means. (Data reproduced from Roffman, Kling, Cassens, Orsulak, Reigle and Schildkraut [1977]: Commun Psychopharmacol 1:195–206.)

$^a p < .001$ compared to control values.

$^b p < .01$ compared to control values.

Thus, by inhibiting the reuptake of norepinephrine, desmethylimipramine and imipramine may increase the norepinephrine available to interact with presynaptic as well as postsynaptic receptors. The slowing of norepinephrine turnover in brain that occurs after acute administration of these tricyclic antidepressant drugs is probably the result of "homeostatic" feedback inhibition, which produces a decrease in locus coeruleus firing rates (16) and possibly also a decrease in the amount of norepinephrine released per nerve impulse. This decrease in the amount of norepinephrine released per nerve impulse may be mediated at least in part by presynaptic alpha-adrenergic receptors and possibly also by other presynaptic receptors (26).

If the release of norepinephrine in brain is decreased after acutely administered imipramine or desmethylimipramine as a result of stimulation of presynaptic alpha-adrenergic receptors, a blockade or a decrease in sensitivity (i.e., subsensitivity) of these receptors may develop gradually during chronic administration of these tricyclic antidepressants, thereby resulting in a gradual increase in norepinephrine turnover in brain (when compared to the slowing of norepinephrine turnover after acute administration of these tricyclic antidepressants). Data supporting this hypothesis have been published recently by Crews and Smith (6) and Svensson and Usdin (33). Since the inhibition of norepinephrine uptake in rat brain produced by desmethylimipramine and imipramine persists after chronic administration of these drugs (18, 26, 30), the gradual increase in norepinephrine turnover that occurs during chronic administration of these tricyclic antidepressant drugs may increase norepinephrine levels in the synapse and at postsynaptic receptors and thus may account for the onset of clinical antidepressant effects after chronic (but not acute) administration of tricyclic antidepressants.

When interpreting these findings, one must consider a number of different factors, including (1) the acute pharmacologic effects of the drug, (2) the direct physiologic consequences of these acute pharmacologic effects, (3) the acute or short-term homeostatic adaptive responses of the organism to these effects, (4) the chronic or long-term pharmacologic effects of the drug, (5) the direct physiologic consequences of these long-term pharmacologic effects, and (6) the adaptive or homeostatic responses of the organism to these long-term effects. When considered in this manner, the data presented suggest hypothetical mechanisms that may account for the intriguing observations that Rapoport and Potter describe in Chapter 8.

These investigators noted a delay in onset of the clinical effects of tricyclic antidepressant drugs in depressed or school-phobic children, just as there is a delay in onset of the clinical antidepressant effects in depressed adults. Moreover, these investigators note the clinical effects of tricyclic antidepressants in school-phobic or depressed children will persist during long-term chronic administration of the drugs. In contrast, Rapoport and Potter note there is no delay in onset of the clinical effects of tricyclic antidepressants in hyperkinetic or in enuretic children and that the clinical effects are often seen following the first dose. However, these investigators indicate there is a "wearing off" (i.e., a diminution or loss) of efficacy in many patients during chronic (2 to 5 week) drug administration. In commenting on these findings, Rapoport and Potter state, "immediate clinical effects of tricyclics seen in children with hyperactivity or enuresis ... are probably mediated by a different mechanism than the delayed clinical effect seen after 2 to 4 weeks in depressed or school-phobic children ..." (Chapter 8, page 108).

The data presented in this chapter on differences between the acute and chronic effects of tricyclic antidepressants on norepinephrine turnover would suggest that in depressed or school-phobic children, just as in depressed adult patients, the gradual increase in norepinephrine turnover that occurs during chronic administration of certain tricyclic antidepressant drugs coupled with their persistent inhibition of norepinephrine uptake may gradually increase levels of norepinephrine at critical receptor sites and, thus, may account for the onset of clinical antidepressant effects occurring only after chronic administration of these tricyclic antidepressants.

In contrast, the immediate clinical effects observed after the first dose of these drugs in hyperkinetic or enuretic children may be due to the inhibition of norepinephrine uptake coupled with the slowing in norepinephrine turnover (reflected in our studies by the decreased rate of disappearance of norepinephrine-^{3}H from brain and the decrease in

MHPG-SO$_4$ levels in brain) that occurs after the acute administration of these tricyclic antidepressant drugs. This hypothesis (that the inhibition of norepinephrine uptake and the consequent slowing in norepinephrine turnover occurring after acute administration of tricyclic antidepressants may account for the clinical effects of tricyclic antidepressants in hyperkinetic children) gains some support from the recent findings of Brown et al. (3), showing that the administration of d-amphetamine to hyperactive boys resulted in a time-dependent decrease in urinary MHPG excretion that appeared to correlate with the clinical behavioral response to treatment with d-amphetamine.

ROLE OF THE BIOCHEMICAL AND PHYSIOLOGIC STATUS OF THE PATIENT IN DETERMINING "CLINICAL" EFFECTS OF TRICYCLIC ANTIDEPRESSANT DRUGS

The observations that tricyclic antidepressant drugs produce an immediate clinical effect in hyperkinetic or enuretic children (with a gradual diminution in the clinical effects during long-term administration), coupled with the observation that tricyclic antidepressants require long-term administration before clinical effects are observed in depressed or school-phobic children, as well as in depressed adults, suggest the pharmacologic mechanisms of action underlying these two types of clinical effects may be quite different and the biochemical pathophysiology underlying these clinical states may also differ. The notion that differences in the underlying biochemical pathophysiology may lead to differences in the clinical effects of tricyclic antidepressant drugs is further exemplified by the studies showing that pretreatment levels of urinary MHPG may provide a biochemical criterion for predicting differential responses to treatment with various tricyclic antidepressant drugs.

The studies of Maas and associates (10) initially showed that patients with "low" levels of urinary MHPG responded more favorably to treatment with imipramine or desmethylimipramine than did patients with higher pretreatment MHPG levels, whereas our early studies suggested patients with "high" pretreatment levels of urinary MHPG responded more favorably to treatment with amitriptyline than did patients with lower MHPG levels (24, 25). Subsequent studies by Beckmann and Goodwin (2) in patients with depressed type unipolar primary affective disorders provided initial confirmation of these findings, but this has not been clearly demonstrated in other studies (5, 20).

Since clinical experience indicates there is an overlap in the clinical spectrum of action of imipramine and amitriptyline (i.e., some depressed patients respond favorably to either of these drugs while others may respond to neither), it seems unlikely that measures of urinary MHPG could provide a nonoverlapping discrimination between imipramine and amitriptyline responders. Rather, these findings suggest that patients with low pretreatment urinary MHPG may be somewhat more likely to respond favorably to imipramine, while patients with higher urinary MHPG would be more likely to respond favorably to amitriptyline.

Corresponding to the suggestion that imipramine and amitriptyline have partially overlapping and partially discrete spectra of clinical antidepressant activities are the neuropharmacologic findings suggesting both similarities and differences in the effects of imipramine and its demethylated metabolite desmethylimipramine versus amitriptyline and its demethylated metabolite nortriptyline on various neurotransmitters, including norepinephrine and serotonin (23). This literature, which has been reviewed recently by Maas (9), suggests that more potent effects on noradrenergic neuronal systems would be observed after administration of imipramine than after administration of amitriptyline.

In this context, it is relevant to present the results of a recent study[1] on the relationship between pretreatment levels of urinary MHPG and response to treatment with maprotiline, a new tetracyclic antidepressant drug that inhibits norepinephrine uptake and is fairly specific for its effects on noradrenergic neuronal systems (11, 12, 34).

In this study (22), we found that depressed patients with "low" pretreatment levels of urinary MHPG were more responsive to treatment with maprotiline than were patients with higher levels of urinary MHPG. More specifically, we found that patients with "low" levels of urinary MHPG required lower doses of maprotiline and responded more rapidly to treatment with maprotiline than did patients with higher pretreatment levels of urinary MHPG.

Patients in the study were started on a 4-week trial of treatment with maprotiline after baseline clinical and biochemical data were collected. To ensure that all patients received an adequate therapeutic trial of maprotiline and that failure to respond to treatment was not due to an inadequate dosage, statistical analyses were performed only on data from those patients who received at least 150 mg/day during the first 2 weeks, unless the patients had shown a favorable clinical response at lower doses. After 2 weeks of treatment with maprotiline, the dosage could be increased at a maximum rate of 50 mg every 3 days, up to a maximum dosage of 300 mg/day.

All patients included in this study met the Research Diagnostic Criteria for major depressive disorder (32), and all but one of the patients met the criteria for endogenous depressive syndrome we have described else-

[1] This study was performed by our collaborative research group, which includes Dr. Alan Schatzberg, Dr. Jonathan Cole, and Dr. William Rohde of McLean Hospital; Dr. Alan Rosenbaum of the Mayo Clinic; and Dr. Paul Orsulak of the Neuropsychopharmacology Laboratory of the Massachusetts Mental Health Center. Results of this study were presented by Dr. Schatzberg at the annual meeting of the American Psychiatric Association held in Chicago in May 1979.

where (28). As shown in Table 4, the patients in this study were well matched for age and baseline Hamilton Depression Rating Scale (HDRS) scores. However, when the clinical data were examined after 2 weeks of treatment with maprotiline, we found that the mean 2-week HDRS scores were significantly lower in patients with low pretreatment urinary MHPG ($\leq$1950 μg/day) than in patients with high pretreatment urinary MHPG (> 1950 μg/day). Moreover, we also found that the mean changes in HDRS scores at 2 weeks and the mean percentage reductions in 2-week HDRS scores from baseline values were significantly greater in patients with low pretreatment urinary MHPG levels than in patients with high pretreatment MHPG levels.

Thus, the findings presented in Table 4 suggest that patients with low pretreatment MHPG levels may respond more rapidly to treatment with relatively low doses of maprotiline than patients with high pretreatment urinary MHPG levels. However, the findings of this study also showed that some patients with high pretreatment levels showed favorable clinical antidepressant response to maprotiline when this drug was administered at higher doses and for longer periods of time.

Although the findings of this study indicate a difference in response patterns to maprotiline in patients with low versus high pretreatment urinary MHPG levels, we cannot draw conclusive biologic inferences from these data or determine clearly the physiologic mechanisms that account for these differences in response patterns. While maprotiline exerts pronounced effects on the uptake of norepinephrine (11, 12, 34), a recent study in animals suggests this drug may also exert some effects on serotonergic neurons (4). Thus, patients with low pretreatment urinary MHPG levels may be more responsive to maprotiline because they have a decrease in central noradrenergic activity, while patients with high pretreatment levels respond only to higher doses of maprotiline, because these doses are required to produce effects on serotonergic neuronal

TABLE 4. Baseline Urinary MHPG and Response to Maprotiline after 2 Weeks

	MHPG $\leq$ 1950 μg/day (n = 11)	MHPG > 1950 μg/day (n = 11)	p
Age (years)	44 ± 4	44 ± 4	NS
Baseline HDRS[a]	33 ± 1	29 ± 2	NS
Two week HDRS[a]	14 ± 2	22 ± 1	< .005
Change in HDRS[a]	18 ± 3	7 ± 2	< .005
Percent reduction in HDRS[a]	54 ± 7	24 ± 5	< .001

Data are expressed as means ± standard errors of the means (Data reproduced from Schatzberg, Rosenbaum, Cole, Rohde, Orsulak, Schildkraut [1979]: Presented at the Annual Meeting of the American Psychiatric Association, Chicago.)

[a]HDRS, Hamilton depression rating scale score.

systems. However, this is probably a gross oversimplification at best, and it is equally possible that further research may show that patients with high pretreatment levels may also have other abnormalities in noradrenergic neuronal systems and that, at higher dose levels, maprotiline may correct these abnormalities by producing further alterations in the metabolism of norepinephrine or in the physiology of noradrenergic neuronal systems (e.g., receptor sensitivity).

CASE STUDY

The following case study illustrates the possible effects of aging on tricyclic antidepressant pharmacokinetics and documents the clinical importance of measuring tricyclic antidepressant levels, particularly in elderly patients. For illustrative purposes, reference will be made to a study of a patient who was seen at Massachusetts Mental Health Center by an alert resident who averted what might have been a tragedy (1).

This patient is a 68-year-old woman with a 12-year history of recurrent depressions that had been treated mainly at other hospitals with electroconvulsive therapy and various tricyclic antidepressant drugs or drug combinations, including amitriptyline in doses up to 200 mg/day. The patient was admitted to the Massachusetts Mental Health Center on February 21, 1979, having been on a dose of 75 mg/day of imipramine. On this dose, she showed a sudden decompensation, and there was some question as to whether she was, in fact, taking the drug as prescribed. As shown in Table 5, at the time of this admission the dose of imipramine was increased to 100 mg/day, and acetophenazine, which had been used previously in this patient's treatment, was added to her drug regimen. When the patient failed to respond after 2 weeks, the resident planned to increase the dose of imipramine, but very wisely decided to measure plasma levels of the tricyclic antidepressants before doing so. He had quite reasonably expected to find low levels, but when the results of the blood levels drawn on March 7 were reported back on March 8, he found much to his surprise that the total tricyclic antidepressant drug level (imipramine plus desmethylimipramine) was 805 ng/ml with a very marked elevation of desmethylimipramine relative to imipramine.

Consequently, on March 8 imipramine was discontinued and another blood sample was obtained for tricyclic antidepressant blood levels on March 9 to confirm whether the previous result could have been a lab error. On March 9 the patient was still found to have a very elevated total tricyclic antidepressant drug level of 696 ng/ml, with desmethylimipramine again being the significantly elevated component. It is noteworthy that physical examination at this point failed to reveal evidence of atropinic toxicity. On March 12, 3 days after imipramine was discontinued, the patient became less agitated, cooperated with nursing staff for the first

TABLE 5. Clinical Utility of Tricyclic Antidepressant (TCA) Blood Levels

Date	Dose (mg/day)	TCA levels (ng/ml)	Clinical condition
2/21	Imi 100 Apz 20	—	Agitated depression
3/7	Imi 100 Apz 20	Imi = 193 Dmi = 612 Total = 805	Agitated depression
3/9	Apz 20	Imi = 174 Dmi = 522 Total = 696	Agitated depression
3/13	Imi 25 Apz 20	—	Improvement
3/20	Imi 25 Apz 20	Imi = 51 Dmi = 201 Total = 252	Discharged improved
3/31	Imi 25—? Apz 20—?	Imi = 23 Dmi = 120 Total = 143	Readmitted agitated depression
4/1	Imi 25/50 qod Apz 20	—	Agitated depression
4/20	Imi 25/50 qod Apz 40	—	Agitated depression
5/2	Imi 25/50 qod Apz 40	Imi = 85 Dmi = 222 Total = 307	Improved

Imi, imipramine; Dmi, desmethylimipramine; Apz, acetophenazine. (Data reproduced from Appelbaum, Vasile, Orsulak, Schildkraut [1979]: Am J Psychiat 136:339–341.)

time, and began to converse socially in an appropriate fashion and to play the piano. Mental status examination revealed a clear sensorium, marked improvement in depressive mood, and no evidence of psychosis. The next day (March 13), treatment with imipramine was resumed in a dose of 25 mg/day. On March 20 the patient was clinically stable and recompensated; her total plasma tricyclic antidepressant blood level was 252 ng/ml (imipramine, 51 ng/ml; desipramine, 201 ng/ml). At this point, the patient was discharged to a nursing home.

The patient was readmitted to Massachusetts Mental Health Center on March 31, because of the reemergence of her depressive syndrome. The total plasma tricyclic antidepressant drug level had fallen to 143 ng/ml (imipramine, 23 ng/ml; desipramine, 120 ng/ml), which is below the usual therapeutic range. Her failure to take the medication as prescribed may have caused this decrease in blood levels and the associated clinical decompensation. On April 1 the dose of imipramine was increased to 25 mg and 50 mg on alternate days. On April 20 the patient still remained unimproved, and the dose of acetophenazine was increased from 20 mg/day to 40 mg/day. One week later the patient recompensated, becoming pleasant and talkative. On May 2 the total tricyclic antidepressant drug level was 307 ng/ml (imipramine, 85 ng/ml; desipramine, 222 ng/ml). The patient was discharged from the Massachusetts Mental Health Center on May 12, and 3 months later she remained in remission while continuing to receive acetophenazine 40 mg/day and imipramine 25 mg/day alternating with 50 mg/day.

During the patient's hospital admission in February and March, routine and accepted clinical practice would have called for an increase in the dosage of imipramine in the face of a failure to respond to a modest dose of 100 mg/day. However, when plasma tricyclic antidepressant drug levels were obtained on March 7, it became clear that these levels were approaching the toxic range and that a decrease in dosage was indicated. In the absence of the determination of tricyclic antidepressant blood levels, neither clinical psychiatric evaluation nor physical examination would have led to the proper psychopharmacologic response.

One of the factors leading to the very high tricyclic antidepressant drug levels observed in this patient may have been the concomitant administration of acetophenazine, since phenothiazines have been reported to inhibit the metabolism of tricyclic antidepressants, particularly of demethylated derivatives such as desipramine (8, 17). However, to reinforce what Friedel notes in Chapter 9, an even more important factor may have been the pharmacokinetic changes that can occur with aging, since this patient, just a few years earlier, had previously tolerated amitriptyline in doses up to 200 mg/day. Thus, pharmacokinetic changes with aging can be extremely important clinically, and assessing plasma levels of tricyclic antidepressants in these patients may not only be of some clinical utility, but in certain cases may even be effectively life saving.

SUMMARY

This chapter has addressed a number of fundamental pharmacodynamic issues that must be considered as we attempt to evaluate the effects of the aging process (from childhood to old age) on the actions of tricyclic antidepressant drugs. The first point discussed was the fact that tricyclic antidepressant drugs have differences as well as similarities in their pharmacodynamic effects and that tricyclic antidepressants produce many other pharmacologic effects in addition to inhibiting the uptake of one or another of the monoamines. Also discussed were some of the differences observed between the effects of acute versus chronic administration of tricyclic antidepressant drugs and how the differences in effects of acute versus chronic administration of these drugs might provide clues with respect to their mechanisms of action in different clinical disorders. Moreover, consideration was given to the role of the biochemical and physiologic status of the patient (in other words, the biochemical pathophysiology of the disorder being treated) in determining the clinical effects that may be observed with one or another of the tricyclic antidepressant drugs. Finally, a brief case study illustrated the pharmacokinetic changes that may occur in association with the aging process or with drug–drug interactions.

REFERENCES AND BIBLIOGRAPHY

1. Appelbaum PS, Vasile RG, Orsulak PJ, Schildkraut JJ (1979): Clinical utility of tricyclic antidepressant blood levels: A case report. Am J Psychiatry 136:339–341.
2. Beckmann H, Goodwin FK (1975): Antidepressant response to tricyclics and urinary MHPG in unipolar patients. Arch Gen Psychiat 32:17–21.
3. Brown GL, Ebert MD, Hunt RD, Rapoport JL (1979): Urinary 3-methoxy-4-hydroxyphenylglycol and homovanillic acid response to d-amphetamine in hyperactive children. Soc of Biological Psychiatrists, Thirty-Fourth Annual Convention and Scientific Program, Chicago, pp 78–79.
4. Carlsson A, Lindqvist M (1978): Effects of antidepressant agents on the synthesis of brain monoamines. J Neural Transm 43:73–91.
5. Coppen A, Rama Rao VA, Ruthven CRJ, Goodwin BL, Sandler M (1979): Urinary 4-hydroxy-3-methoxy-phenylglycol is not a predictor for clinical response to amitriptyline in depressive illness. Psychopharmacology 64:95–97.
6. Crews FT, Smith CB (1978): Presynaptic alpha-receptor subsensitivity after long-term antidepressant treatment. Science 202:322–324.
7. Glowinski J, Axelrod J (1966): Effects of drugs on disposition of H^3-norepinephrine in rat brain. Pharmacol Rev 18:775–785.
8. Gram LF, Overo KF (1972): Drug interaction: Inhibitory effect of neuroleptics on metabolism of tricyclic antidepressants in man. Br Med J 1:463–465.
9. Maas JW (1978): Clinical and biochemical heterogeneity of depressive disorders. Ann Intern Med 88:556–663.
10. Maas JW, Fawcett JA, Dekirmenjian H (1972): Catecholamine metabolism, depressive illness, and drug response. Arch Gen Psychiatry 26:252–262.
11. Maitre L, Staehelin M, Bein JJ (1971): Blockade of noradrenaline uptake by 34276a, a new antidepressant drug. Biochem Pharmacol 20:2169–2186.
12. Maitre L, Waldmeier PC, Greengrass PM, Jackel J, Sedlacek S, Delini-Stula A (1975): Maprotline—Its position as an antidepressant in the light of recent neuropharmacological and neurobiochemical findings. J Int Med Res (Suppl 2) 3:1–15.
13. Meek JL, Neff NH (1973): The rate of formation of 3-methoxy-4-hydroxyphenyleneglycol sulfate in brain as an index of the rate of formation of norepinephrine. J Pharmacol Exp Ther 184:570–575.
14. Nielsen M (1975): The influence of desipramine and amitriptyline on the accumulation of ^3H-noradrenaline and its two major metabolites formed from ^3H-tyrosine in the rat brain. J Pharm Pharmacol 27:206–209.

15. Nielsen M, Eplov L, Scheel-Kruger J (1975): The effects of amitriptyline, desipramine and imipramine on the *in vivo* brain synthesis of ^{3}H-noradrenaline from ^{3}H-1-dopa in the rat. Psychopharmacologia 41:249–254.

16. Nyback HV, Walters JR, Aghajanian GK, Roth RH (1975): Tricyclic antidepressants: Effects on the firing rate of brain noradrenergic neurons. Eur J Pharmacol 32:302–312.

17. Olivier-Martin R, Marzin D, Buschsenschutz E, Pichot P, Boissier J (1975): Concentrations plasmatiques de l'imipramine et de la desméthylimipramine et l'effect antidepresseur au cours d'un traitement controlé. Psychopharmacologia 41:187–195.

18. Roffler-Tarlov S, Schildkraut JJ (1971): Norepinephrine (NE) content and turnover in rat brain regions after acute and chronic treatment with desmethylimipramine (DMI). Fed Proc 30:381.

19. Roffman M, Kling MA, Cassens G, Orsulak PJ, Reigle TG, Schildkraut JJ (1977): The effects of acute and chronic administration of tricyclic antidepressants on MHPG-SO$_4$ in rat brain. Commun Psychopharmacol 1:195–206.

20. Sacchetti E, Allaria E, Negri F, Biondi PA, Smeraldi E, Cazzullo CL (1979): 3-Methoxy-4-hydroxyphenylglycol and primary depression: Clinical and pharmacological considerations. Biol Psychiatry 14:473–484.

21. Schanberg SM, Schildkraut JJ, Breese GR, Kopin IJ (1968): Metabolism of normetanephrin H^3 in rat brain: Identification of conjugated 3-methoxy-4-hydroxyphenylglycol as the major metabolite. Biochem Pharmacol 17:247–254.

22. Schatzberg A, Rosenbaum A, Cole J, Rohde W, Orsulak PJ, Schildkraut JJ (1979): Preliminary studies of maprotiline. Presented at the Annual Meeting of the American Psychiatric Association, Chicago.

23. Schildkraut JJ (1970): Neuropsychopharmacology and the Affective Disorders. Boston, Little, Brown.

24. Schildkraut JJ (1973): Norepinephrine metabolites as biochemical criteria for classifying depressive disorders and predicting responses to treatment: Preliminary findings. Am J Psychiatry 130:695–699.

25. Schildkraut JJ (1974): Biochemical criteria for classifying depressive disorders and predicting responses to pharmacotherapy: Preliminary findings from studies of norepinephrine metabolism. Pharmakopsychiatr Neuropsychopharmakol 7:98–107.

26. Schildkraut JJ (1975): Norepinephrine metabolism after short- and long-term administration of tricyclic antidepressant drugs and electroconvulsive shock. In Mandell, AJ ed: Neurobiological Mechanisms of Adaptation and Behavior, New York, Raven Press, pp 137–153.

27. Schildkraut JJ, Dodge GA, Logue MA (1969): Effects of tricyclic antidepressants on the uptake and metabolism of intracisternally administered norepinephrine-H^3 in rat brain. J Psychiatric Res 7:29–34.

28. Schildkraut JJ, Orsulak PJ, Schatzberg AF, Gudeman JE, Cole JO, Rohde WA, LaBrie RA (1978): Toward a biochemical classification of depressive disorders I: Differences in urinary MHPG and other catecholamine metabolites in clinically defined subtypes of depressions. Arch Gen Psychiatry 35:1427–1433.

29. Schildkraut JJ, Schanberg SM, Breese GR, Kopin IJ (1967): Norepinephrine metabolism and drugs used in the affective disorders: A possible mechanism of action. Am J Psychiatry 124:600–608.

30. Schildkraut JJ, Winokur A, Applegate CW (1970): Norepinephrine turnover and metabolism in rat brain after long-term administration of imipramine. Science 168:867–869.

31. Schildkraut JJ, Winokur A, Draskoczy PR, Hensle JH (1971): Changes in norepinephrine turnover in rat brain during chronic administration of imipramine and protriptyline: a possible explanation for the delay in onset of clinical antidepressant effects. Am J Psychiatry 27:1032–1039.

32. Spitzer RL, Endicott J, Robins E (1978): Research diagnostic criteria (RDC) for a selected group of functional disorders, New York State Psychiatric Institute, 3rd ed, 1 February.

33. Svensson TH, Usdin T (1978): Feedback inhibition of brain noradrenalin neurons by tricyclic antidepressants. Science 202:1089–1091.

34. Waldmeier PC, Baumann P, Greengrass PM, Maitre L (1976): Effects of clomipramine and other tricyclic antidepressants on biogenic amine uptake and turnover. Postgrad Med J (Suppl 3) 52:33–39.

11

MONOAMINE OXIDASE INHIBITORS AND THE ELDERLY

Donald S. Robinson

Our interest in monoamine oxidase inhibitors (MAOIs) began several years ago with the first of a series of controlled clinical trials of phenelzine treatment of outpatients with depressive illness (25). The two initial placebo-controlled trials demonstrated antidepressant activity of phenelzine in depression (16, 18, 25). Furthermore, there appeared to be no evidence of significant therapeutic effect of phenelzine until platelet MAO was inhibited at least 80% from the pretreatment control value.

Currently we are engaged in a double-blind comparison study of phenelzine and the tricyclic antidepressant amitriptyline in depression (19). The major purpose of this study is to define the clinical spectra of these two antidepressants and to identify differential therapeutic effects. In this outpatient trial, plasma levels of each drug and certain of their metabolite levels are being serially measured. The relationships of drug level to clinical outcome and side effects are also being assessed in this study, in which patients receive a fixed dose of antidepressant drug over a 6 week treatment period.

Although these various phenelzine studies were not designed prospectively to test for age relationships, we have examined data retrospectively from these trials to see whether age might be an important biologic variable influencing drug response or pharmacologic effects of either antidepressant agent. For this presentation emphasis is placed on the

From the Department of Pharmacology, Marshall University, School of Medicine, Huntington, West Virginia.

Supported in part by grant R01 MH 27836 from the National Institute of Mental Health.

relationship of age and the MAOI, phenelzine, about which more is known that the other MAOIs.

Age relationships are interesting for several reasons in psychopharmacology, especially with antidepressant drug therapy. So far as I can tell, therapeutic response to MAOIs has not been studied previously for evidence of significant associations with aging. Concern has been expressed by some that MAOIs may be less well tolerated by older patients, or may actually have a greater toxic liability in the elderly. Certainly, the more popular and widely used tricyclic antidepressants (TCAs) do present significant problems in the elderly, both with respect to a predisposition to troublesome side effects (4), as well as the recently recognized decreased metabolism and clearance of TCAs with advancing age (15). Finally, there is some reason to speculate that MAOIs might possess special efficacy or therapeutic advantage in older patients, based on the observations of increased MAO activity with aging observed in several human tissues including brain and platelet (22).

AGE AND MONOAMINE METABOLISM

It is at least of some passing interest that the specific activity of MAO in a variety of tissues tends to increase with age throughout adulthood. This appears to be a generalized phenomenon in human tissues. In 1971, in collaboration with Dr. John Davis, we obtained for study hindbrains from patients who died from a variety of causes. The results of this investigation showed that mean MAO activity in hindbrain increased significantly with age, with roughly a twofold difference between young adults and persons over 60 years of age (23).

In a subsequent study we examined MAO activity in homogenates prepared from several brain regions in a series of 39 human brains obtained at autopsy (26). MAO activity correlated positively with age in all brain areas and with both benzylamine and tryptamine as substrates. During adolescence there is a second peak in enzyme activity that has been observed with both brain and platelet MAO (26). Thus, there appears to be a nadir in brain and platelet MAO activity occurring between 20 and 40 years of age, followed by a progressive rise in enzyme activity up to age 80 years. Platelet MAO activities of outpatients with depression from our clinical trials similarly show this pattern, representing a replication of previous findings of a significant age correlation as well as sex difference in enzyme activity (Figure 1). Other investigators have also reported similar age trends and sex differences in both platelet and brain MAO activity (7, 9, 13, 14, 22, 23, 26).

Further, in a regional postmortem study of monoamine metabolism in human brain, a decline in norepinephrine (NE) levels (μg/g tissue) in

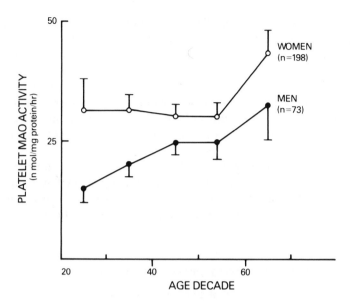

FIGURE 1. Platelet monoamine oxidase (MAO) levels of men and women outpatients with depression. Mean MAO activity (n mol/mg protein/hour ± SEM) per decade, with benzylamine as substrate, is shown for each sex.

older subjects was observed in most areas examined (26). However, the concentrations of the indoleamine, serotonin, did not seem to fluctuate with age. The pattern of age-related regional decreases in brain NE content could reflect either a loss of adrenergic neurons and synaptic terminals, or an intrinsic change in neuronal synthesis, degradation and turnover of NE, or both. Suggestive evidence exists that the increased MAO activity in aged brains could reside primarily in postsynaptic or extraneuronal tissues rather than in adrenergic neurons. Experiments using 6-hydroxydopamine as an investigative tool are consistent with this hypothesis (1, 3), and further work needs to be done to elucidate the patterns of cellular and subcellular distribution of MAO in CNS tissues.

Recently we reported another biologic change with implications for altered CNS catecholamine metabolism with aging. Using a recently developed and sensitive assay technique, pterin cofactor activity was measured in the cerebrospinal fluid (CSF) of normal subjects and patients with various degenerative diseases of the basal ganglia (24). Biopterin, the pteridine cofactor catalyzing the hydroxylation of phenylalanine and tyrosine in the synthesis of dopamine and NE, may exist in rate-limiting concentrations in vivo in neuronal tissues in brain, at least in striatum (12). In a large series of normals a significant negative correlation of age and pteridine cofactor activity in CSF was found (24). Patients with degenerative diseases involving the basal ganglia have consistently lower levels of CSF pterin cofactor activity than normal elderly subjects. In these patients CSF cofactor activity also correlated negatively with age. These data provide additional evidence of biologic changes of aging that may contribute to a trend for decreased catecholamine neurotransmitter levels in the elderly. In Chapter 3 Levine and coworkers discuss in more detail the relationships of age to CSF levels of cofactor activity in both health and psychiatric and neurologic illness.

All the studies cited above point toward some form of impairment of monoamine metabolism as a concomitant of aging. They have important implications with respect to underlying biochemical etiologies of psychiatric and cardiovascular disorders of aging as well as specific treatments for the elderly.

AGE AND RESPONSE TO ANTIDEPRESSANT DRUGS

After stratifying for age we analyzed the characteristics of antidepressant drug responders. In the phenelzine-amitriptyline trial in progress (19) and the previous phenelzine-placebo clinical trials (18, 25) drug response rates were computed by inclusion of all patients who started the drug treatment protocol including drug failures who became dropouts. Table 1 shows the fraction of patients demonstrating favorable antidepressant response as determined by global evaluation (blind rating by psychiatrist) after 6 weeks' treatment with either amitriptyline 150 mg or phenelzine 60 mg daily. For the first 5 days of treatment, half dosage of each drug was administered to minimize initial side effects. The full dose was administered for the remainder of the 6 week period of drug therapy. For both

TABLE 1. Response Rate to Amitriptyline and Phenelzine Treatment as a Function of Age in Outpatients with Depression[a]

Age (yr)	Amitriptyline		Phenelzine	
	Response rate (%)	n	Response rate (%)[b]	n
<30	50	18	26	31
30 to 45	57	28	54	67
45 to 60	25	16	56	36
>60	60	5	69	13

[a]After an initial 1-week drug washout period, outpatients with significant depressive symptomatology were treated as part of a double-blind controlled clinical trial for 6 weeks with either amitriptyline 150 mg/day or phenylzine 60 mg/day (18, 19, 25). Percent patients (includes completors and dropouts) who showed significant improvement by global rating (blind) of psychiatrist is shown.

[b]Responders to phenelzine were significantly older than nonresponders by Wilcoxon rank order test ($p < .01$).

the amitriptyline and phenelzine treatment groups there was a comparable dropout rate of approximately 20%. Inclusion of dropouts in the data analysis accounts for the apparent lower response rates to antidepressant drug, i.e., around 60% or fewer patients showing significant improvement by the sixth week, depending on age stratum. The general experience in the psychopharmacologic literature reveals that drug response rates calculated by disregarding dropouts range anywhere from 55 to 75%, depending on the patient sample, type of antidepressant drug, treatment setting, etc. (10).

Response to amitriptyline did not show a consistent trend across age strata (Table 1). The apparent poor response to amitriptyline in the 45 to 60 year stratum most likely occurred by chance and is attributable to the small cell size. On the other hand, in phenelzine-treated patients there is a progressive and statistically significant trend with advancing age for a higher probability of favorable antidepressant response. Curiously (and rather unexpectedly) there was a somewhat low response rate to phenelzine in patients under 30 years of age. However, the phenelzine response rate was highest (nearly 70%) in patients over age 60 years. The number of patients in each cell are larger for phenelzine than for amitriptyline because the results shown in Table 1 include phenelzine-treated patients from previous placebo-controlled clinical trials (18, 25) whose experimental design was similar to the amitriptyline-phenelzine study still in progress (19). Since the number of patients over 60 years is still relatively small, we must interpret with caution the apparently more favorable response rate to phenelzine in the elderly patient. Obviously these can be considered only preliminary findings which await verification and require replication. Nevertheless, the positive association of age and enhanced probability of favorable response to phenelzine is statistically significant (Wilcoxon rank order test, $p < .01$) and belies the unsubstantiated fear that older patients if anything might tolerate MAOIs poorly.

AGE AND ANTIDEPRESSANT DRUG SIDE EFFECTS

We examined side effects in relation to patient age for each antidepressant drug treatment (Table 2). During the clinical trial, patient side effects were routinely elicited and rated every 2 weeks using a checklist administered by the psychiatrist. The mean number of side effects reported per patient was slightly greater with amitriptyline than with phenelzine treatment. Unexpectedly, there was also a significantly higher incidence of drug side effects reported by amitriptyline-treated patients younger than age 50 years than in those over age 50 or in patients treated with phenelzine, irrespective of age.

Table 3 lists the three most common side effects according to age encountered with amitriptyline or phenelzine treatment in our outpatient

TABLE 2. Numbers of Side Effects Reported by Patients During Treatment
with Amitriptyline or Phenelzine

Age (yrs)	Amitriptyline		Phenelzine			
	Mean ± SEM	n	Mean ± SEM	n	t	p
<50	3.4 ± 0.3^a	42	2.5 ± 0.2	46	2.49	<.02
>50	2.8 ± 0.6	13	2.2 ± 0.3	12	0.73	NS
Total	3.22 ± 0.20^a	55	2.47 ± 0.22	58	2.47	<.02

[a]Mean number of side effects reported per patient attributable to drug treatment with 150 mg/day amitriptyline is significantly greater than with phenelzine 60 mg/day (Student's t test two sided).

sample. Interestingly, sedation was reported almost as frequently with phenelzine as amitriptyline treatment, although it was generally less severe and troublesome with the MAOI. Sedation due to amitriptyline tended to be more prominent during the first 10 days of therapy, even though the drug was administered at half-dosage for the first 5 days. Tolerance to this side effect, attributable to the well known central anticholinergic and antihistaminic properties of amitriptyline, generally develops within several days and was not any different in older than in younger patients.

The most frequently encountered side effect was dry mouth, associated with amitriptyline treatment (Table 3). Dry mouth is also fairly regularly reported by phenelzine-treated patients but generally is less pronounced. It is unlikely that reports of dry mouth associated with phenelzine therapy

TABLE 3. Most Common Side Effects Reported with Amitriptyline and
Phenelzine Treatment as a Function of Age[a]

Age (yrs)	Percent sedation		Percent dry mouth		Percent orthostatic dizziness	
	Ami	Phe	Ami	Phe	Ami	Phe
≤ 50	60^b	48	90^c	52	43	50
	(25/42)	(22/46)	(38/42)	(24/46)	(18/42)	(23/46)
> 50	54	50	54	42	31	67
	(7/13)	(6/12)	(7/13)	(5/12)	(4/13)	(8/12)
Total	58	48	82	50	40	54
	(32/55)	(28/58)	(45/55)	(29/58)	(22/55)	(31/58)

[a]Patients treated with either amitriptyline (Ami) 150 mg/day or phenelzine (Phe) 60 mg/day for 6 weeks.

[b]Percent of patients who reported sedation as a side effect at any time during the study.

[c]Proportion of patients reporting dry mouth is significantly greater in younger than in older amitriptyline patients or in phenelzine-treated patients of all ages by chi squares test ($p < .02$).

are artifactual, because of the side-effect rating system employed in this study, which recorded pretreatment symptoms as well as subsequent drug side effects. Again, patients under age 50 years receiving amitriptyline experienced significantly greater incidence of dry mouth than either older patients treated with amitriptyline or phenelzine-treated patients.

Another frequent and potentially troublesome side effect of antidepressant drug treatment is orthostatic hypotension. Table 4 lists mean standing blood pressures, stratified by age above and below 50 years, before and after 6 weeks of treatment with either amitriptyline or phenelzine. Amitriptyline treatment produced little change in standing systolic or diastolic blood pressure, irrespective of age. Nor did the older amitriptyline-treated patients report posturally related dizziness more frequently than younger patients (Table 3). On the other hand, phenelzine treatment did produce a significant decrease in standing blood pressure in some patients (an average decrease of approximately 28 mm Hg systolic and 15 mm Hg diastolic pressure in patients over age 50 years). Eight of the 12 phenelzine-treated patients over age 50 years did experience some orthostatic symptoms. Because of this small sample, statistical significance was not achieved.

This effect of drug on blood pressure was apparent during the first weeks of phenelzine treatment, and did not change or ameliorate with continued treatment. Interestingly, this hypotensive effect of phenelzine treatment was not a limiting side effect, even in older patients. Although orthostatic dizziness was reported more frequently by the older

TABLE 4. Changes in Standing Blood Pressures: Effects of Antidepressant Drug Treatment and Age[a]

Drug	Age (yrs)			
	≤50		>50	
	Before	During	Before	During
Amitriptyline	124 ± 15	121 ± 14	130 ± 17	130 ± 12
	85 ± 10	87 ± 12	88 ± 7	90 ± 8
		$(n = 43)$		$(n = 14)$
Phenelzine	125 ± 15	118 ± 16	144 ± 20	116 ± 27[b,c]
	82 ± 10	82 ± 10	89 ± 13	74 ± 17
		$(n = 46)$		$(n = 12)$

[a]Mean standing blood pressures ± SEM before and after 6 weeks of treatment with either amitriptyline 150 mg/day or phenelzine 60 mg/day.

[b]Change in blood pressure from pretreatment value after 6 weeks of phenelzine treatment is significant ($p < .01$, paired t test).

[c]Orthostatic drop in systolic blood pressure (change from sitting to standing BP) due to phenelzine treatment is significant in patients over 50 years of age ($p < .05$; paired t test).

patients treated with phenelzine (Table 3), it was not a particularly severe or troublesome symptom.

We examined whether this side effect of orthostatic dizziness on rapidly assuming the upright position required discontinuance or reducing the dose of phenelzine. It was rarely necessary to discontinue phenelzine treatment or to modify the dose because of faintness. Interestingly, our findings are similar to those reported by Glassman et al. (6) with imipramine, in that patients who experience a substantial drop in blood pressure with antidepressant drug treatment usually do not require a dose change. Nor was there a significantly higher dropout rate from drug treatment in the phenelzine-treated group, even among older patients. The symptom of postural dizziness associated with orthostatic hypotension is something to which those patients who experience this side effect become progressively more tolerant with continued phenelzine administration, as has been reported with imipramine (6).

RELATIONSHIP OF PLASMA DRUG LEVELS TO CLINICAL EFFECTS AS A FUNCTION OF AGE

We examined which pharmacologic measurements might be associated with drug-induced blood pressure changes during either amitriptyline or phenelzine treatment. Unlike Glassman et al. (6) we did find significant relationships between plasma levels of both phenelzine and amitriptyline and orthostatic drop in blood pressure (Table 5). However, the degree of platelet MAO inhibition did not correlate with decrease in blood pressure

TABLE 5. Orthostatic Drop in Blood Pressure with Antidepressant Treatment: Relationship to Plasma Drug Concentrations and Platelet Monoamine Oxidase Inhibition

Treatment group	Correlation of orthostatic drop in blood pressure and plasma drug level or percent MAO inhibitions (Pearson r)	
	Systolic BP	Diastolic BP
Amitriptyline ($n = 53$ patients)[a]		
Plasma AMI	+.31[b]	+.25
Plasma NT	+.31[b]	+.27[b]
Phenelzine ($n = 54$ patients)[a]		
Plasma phenelzine	+.34[c]	+.46[c]
Percent MAO inhibition	+.08	+.13

[a]Plasma amitriptyline (AMI) and nortriptyline (NT) concentrations after 6 weeks of treatment with amitriptyline, or plasma phenelzine concentrations after 6 weeks treatment with phenelzine are correlated with the orthostatic change in blood pressure from sitting to standing position.

[b]$p < .05$

[c]$p < .01$

on standing (Table 5). These correlations are significant but generally of low order, indicating that plasma drug levels account for only a small portion of the total variance. Nevertheless, these findings represent one of the few instances in which significant correlation has been found between plasma levels and clinical effect of antidepressant drug.

Plasma phenelzine levels have been found to have significant age relationships. Using a recently developed sensitive gas liquid chromatograph (GLC) assay for phenelzine (2), we measured drug levels in patients receiving this drug in the comparison trial of phenelzine and amitriptyline (19). In depressed outpatients treated with 60-mg/day plasma phenelzine concentration (mean) showed a progressive rise over the 6 weeks of drug treatment. It is possible that steady-state plasma phenelzine levels may not have been reached by the sixth week of treatment (Table 6). Plasma phenelzine concentrations were exceedingly low during the initial weeks of treatment, presumably because of the unique pharmacokinetics of this "suicide" drug, which acts as a noncompetitive inhibitor of tissue and platelet MAO by binding irreversibly to the enzyme. Presumably this drug has a high affinity for active sites on the enzyme, and phenelzine concentrations in extracellular fluids are not in equilibrium with receptor-bound drug. Studies are now in progress to define the pharmacokinetics of phenelzine in human beings.

Older patients tend to have higher phenelzine plasma levels than younger patients, most marked during the first 2 weeks of treatment (Table 6). This correlation of plasma phenelzine levels with age is independent of body weight. The correlation of plasma level phenelzine with platelet MAO inhibition is of particular interest, since the association became

TABLE 6. Relationship of Plasma Phenelzine Concentration to Several Clinical and Pharmacologic Variables[a]

Time (wk)	Mean phenelzine concentration in plasma (ng/ml)	Correlation coefficient[b]			
		Age (r)	Global improvement (r)	Percent MAO inhibition (platelet)	
				Benzylamine substrate (tau)	Tryptamine substrate (tau)
2	0.67	$+.32^c$	$-.06$	0.0	0.21^c
4	0.81	$+.16$	$+.15$	$+.14$	$+.46^d$
6	1.29	$+.14$	$+.26^c$	$+.24^c$	$+.30^d$

[a]43 patients in amitriptyline controlled clinical trial treated with phenelzine 60 mg/day for 6 weeks.
[b]Correlation (Pearson r or Kendall tau) with plasma phenelzine concentration significance.
[c]$p < .05$
[d]$p < .01$

progressively greater with continuing treatment. The higher phenelzine plasma levels in older patients may reflect a decreased apparent volume of distribution of phenelzine in the elderly, which has been reported for other psychopharmacologic agents such as diazepam (11).

After 6 weeks of phenelzine treatment, plasma phenelzine levels also correlate with improvement on several major symptom scales of the structured depression interview, including the 17-item Hamilton Depression Scale ($r = .33$, $p < .01$). The tendency for somewhat higher plasma phenelzine levels in the older patients and the greater clinical response to MAOI in these patients might reflect a slower rate of phenelzine metabolism and clearance.

ACETYLATOR PHENOTYPE, DRUG RESPONSE, AND AGE

The rate of drug acetylation in the phenelzine-treated patients was examined. Acetylator phenotyping was carried out in 40 patients from our phenelzine-controlled clinical trials using sulfapyridine according to the method of Price-Evans (17). This acetylator phenotyping identified 25 slow and 15 fast acetylators. Interestingly, no relationship was found between rate of drug acetylation and clinical improvement or percent platelet MAO inhibition. Also, rate of drug acetylation did not appear to be influenced by aging. These findings do not support the suggestion that acetylation is a major determinant of phenelzine metabolism in human beings; also it appears that the nonmicrosomal enzyme, acetyltransferase, like MAO does not diminish in activity with aging. This is consistent with a recent study by Farah et al. (5), who found isoniazid half-lives to be unaffected by age, while acetanilid half-lives were prolonged significantly in the elderly.

SUMMARY

This paper reviewed recent pharmacokinetic, biologic, and clinical data relating to aging and the antidepressant drugs phenelzine and amitriptyline. The MAO-inhibiting drugs have been relatively unstudied in the aged. Considerably more work is required to delineate the therapeutic role of the MAOIs in elderly populations as well as in different diagnostic categories and symptom complexes. There is evidence that biotransformation of phenelzine, as in the tricyclic antidepressant drugs, is slowed in the elderly, and modified doses should be employed in some cases. Phenelzine may have enhanced efficacy in the older patient. It appears that phenelzine is reasonable well tolerated and clinically effective in patients over age 60 years. This may relate to the higher tissue MAO activity associated with the aging process. The relative intolerance to tricyclic antidepressants in the elderly may also favor increased use of MAOIs in this population for the treatment of depression and pseudodementia. The data presented herein can only be considered preliminary since limited numbers of patients over age 60 years have been studied. The highest response rate to phenelzine in our outpatient study has been in the older patient group while somewhat surprisingly, it was lowest in the group under 30 years of age.

Orthostatic drop in blood pressure with phenelzine 60 mg/day is most prominent in patients over 50 years of age. While this is a common side effect encountered in the elderly patient, it has not been especially troublesome. It has been necessary to discontinue phenelzine or reduce its dosage only rarely for this indication. A pattern of higher plasma phenelzine levels in patients over 50 years of age suggests decreased drug biotransformation and metabolism with aging as has been previously reported with the tricyclic antidepressants.

This research was carried out in collaboration with Dr. Alexander Nies, Department of Psychiatry, Marshall University School of Medicine, Huntington, West Virginia, Thomas B. Cooper, Rockland Research Institute, Orangeburg, New York, and Dr. C. Lewis Ravaris, Department of Psychiatry, Eastern Carolina School of Medicine, Greenville, North Carolina. The invaluable assistance of Diantha Howard, Derek Nicoll, Mary Varese, and Sally Roberts is gratefully acknowledged.

REFERENCES AND BIBLIOGRAPHY

1. Breese GR, Traylor TD (1970): Effect of 6-hydroxydopamine on brain norepinephrine and dopamine: Evidence for selective degeneration of catecholamine neurons. J Pharmacol Exp Ther 174:413–420.

2. Cooper TB, Robinson, DS, Nies A (1978): Phenelzine measurement in human plasma: A sensitive GCL-ECD procedure. Commun Psychopharmacol 2:502–512.

3. Cooper JR, Bloom FE, Roth RH (1978): Catecholamines I: General aspects. In JR Louper, FE Bloom, RH Roth, eds: The Biochemical Basis of Neuropharmacology, 3rd ed. New York, Oxford University Press, p 145.

4. Davies RK, Tucker GJ, Harrow M, Detre TP (1971): Confusional episodes and antidepressant medication. Am J Psychiatry 128:95–99.

5. Farah F, Taylor W, Rawlins MD, James O (1977): Hepatic drug acetylation and oxidation: Effects of aging in man. Br Med J 2:155–156.

6. Glassman AH, Biggs JT, Giardina EV, Kantor SJ, Perel JM, Davies M (1979): Clinical characteristics of imipramine-induced orthostatic hypotension. Lancet 1:468–472.

7. Gottfries CG, Oreland L, Wiberg A, Winblad B (1975): Lowered monoamine oxidase activity in brains from alcoholic suicides. J Neurochem 25:667–673.

8. Greenblatt DJ, Allen MD, Shader RI (1978): Factors influencing diazepam pharmacokinetics: Age, sex, and liver disease. Int J Clin Pharmacol Biopharm 16:177–179.

9. Grote SS, Moses, SG, Robins E, Hudgens RW, Croninger AB (1974): A study of selected catecholamine metabolizing enzymes: A comparison of depressive suicides and alcoholic suicides with controls. J Neurochem 23:791–802.

10. Klein DF, Davis JM (1969): Diagnosis and Drug Treatment of Psychiatric Disorders. Baltimore, Williams & Wilkins.

11. Klotz U, Avanti GR, Hoyumpa A, Schenker S, Wilkinson GR (1975): The effects of age and liver disease on the disposition and elimination of diazepam in man. J Clin Invest 55:347–359.

12. Lovenberg W, Victor WJ (1974): Regulation of tryptophan and tyrosine hydroxylase. Life Sci 14:2337–2353.

13. Mann J (1978): Altered platelet monoamine oxidase activity in untreated depression. Presented at the 11th Congress of the Collegium Internationale Neuro-Psychopharmacologium, Vienna, 9–14 July.

14. Murphy DL, Belmaker R, Wyatt RJ (1974): Monoamine oxidase in schizophrenia and other behavioral disorders J Psychiatr Res 11:221–247.

15. Nies A, Robinson DS, Friedman MJ, Green R, Cooper TB, Ravaris CL, Ives JO (1977): Relationship between age and tricyclic antidepressant plasma levels. Am J Psychiatry 134:790–793.

16. Nies A, Robinson DS, Lamborn KR, Ravaris CL, Ives JO (1974): The efficacy of the MAO inhibitor, phenelzine: Dose effects and prediction of response. In JR Boissier, H Hippius, P Pichot, eds: Neuropsychopharmacology, Excerpta Medica International Congress Series No. 359. Excerpta Medica, Amsterdam. pp 765–770.

17. Price-Evans DA (1969): An improved and simplified method of detecting the acetylator phenotype. J Med Genet 6:405–407.

18. Ravaris, CL, Nies A, Robinson DS, Ives JO, Lamborn KR, Korson L (1976): A multiple-dose, controlled study of phenelzine in depression-anxiety states. Arch Gen Psychiatry 33:347–350.

19. Ravaris CL, Robinson SD, Ives JO, Nies A, Bartlett D (1980): A comparison of phenelzine and amitriptyline in the treatment of depression. Arch Gen Psychiatry 37:1075–1080.

20. Robinson DS (1975): Changes in monoamine oxidase and monoamines with human development and aging. Fed Proc 34:103–107.

21. Robinson DS (1979): Age-related factors affecting drug metabolism and clinical response. In Nandy K, ed: Geriatric Psychopharmacology, New York, Elsevier North Holland.

22. Robinson DS, Davis JM, Nies A, Colburn RW, Davis JN, Bourne HR, Bunney WE, Shaw, DM, Coppen, AJ (1972): Ageing, monoamines, and monoamine-oxidase levels. Lancet 1:290–291.

23. Robinson DS, Davis JM, Nies A, Ravaris CL, Sylwester D (1971): Relation of sex and aging to monoamine oxidase activity of human brain, plasma and platelets. Arch Gen Psychiatry 24:536–539.

24. Robinson DS, Levine R, Williams A, Statham NS (1978): Hydroxylase cofactor in human CSF—An index of central aminergic function. Psychopharmacol Bull 14:49–51.

25. Robinson DS, Nies A, Ravaris CL, Lamborn KR (1973): The monoamine oxidase inhibitor, phenelzine, in the treatment of depressive-anxiety states. Arch Gen Psychiatry 29:407–413.

26. Robinson DS, Sourkes TL, Nies A, Harris LS, Spector S, Bartlett DL, Kaye IS (1977): Monoamine metabolism in human brain. Arch Gen Psychiatry 34:89–92.

12

AGE-RELATED CHANGES IN LITHIUM PHARMACOKINETICS

Robert F. Prien

Lithium research is one of the most active areas in psychopharmacology and biologic psychiatry. There are more than 6000 reports in the literature on the biologic, pharmacologic, and psychologic effects of lithium. This report focuses on only selected aspects of the pharmacology of lithium, namely, the relationship between pharmacokinetics and age. Before discussing age-related changes, it is useful to review some of the pharmacokinetic principles underlying lithium therapy.

GENERAL PHARMACOKINETICS

Absorption and Distribution

Lithium is absorbed rapidly following all routes of administration: oral, subcutaneous, intramuscular, and intraperitoneal. Oral administration is the only route used clinically. The lithium ion is well-absorbed from the gastrointestinal tract and passes directly from the bloodstream to the tissues without evidence of protein or plasma binding. Peak plasma levels occur within 2 to 4 hours following a single dose (2). The biologic half-life in individuals with normal renal function varies from 8 to 26 hours (2, 14). In patients with impaired renal function, the half-life is appreciably longer. Equilibrium between the amount of drug absorbed and eliminated (steady state) is established completely after about six to seven half-lives; 90% of the steady state level is reached after approximately three half-lives (3).

From the Psychopharmacology Research Branch, National Institute of Mental Health, Bethesda, Maryland.

A. Raskin, D. S. Robinson, and J. Levine, eds., Age and the Pharmacology of Psychoactive Drugs.

Thus, equilibrium occurs 2 to 7 days after initiating therapy in patients with normal renal function.

The average apparent volume of distribution of lithium corresponds to 50 to 90% of body weight, with marked interindividual variation (14, 18). The volume of distribution range of 0.7 to 1.2 liters/kg seen in the population reflects total body water intracellularly and in saliva that is considerably greater than plasma and indicative of an active transport process.

The concentration of lithium in plasma is used to monitor therapeutic dosage. On the average, a dose of 300 mg of lithium carbonate increases the lithium level by 0.2 to 0.4 mEq/liter (27). Studies indicate that plasma lithium levels of 0.9 to 1.4 mEq/liter are adequate for the treatment of most patients with acute mania (23). Levels of 0.6 to 1.2 mEq/liter are recommended for maintenance treatment (1, 20). The milligram dosage required to achieve a given steady-state plasma level of lithium may vary by as much as 400% among physically healthy individuals (28).

The plasma lithium level is not a completely accurate index of the concentration of lithium in all tissues. The rate of uptake of lithium into various tissues is not uniform. Lithium is rapidly absorbed by the kidney and the spleen, but penetrates more slowly into bone, muscle, and brain (21). In addition, tissues seem to differ markedly in their capacity to concentrate lithium. The lithium concentration in spinal fluid is about one-fourth of that in blood serum, while the thyroid concentration is two to five times greater (3, 13). The lithium concentration in whole brain is approximately the same as in blood serum.

Excretion

More than 95% of ingested lithium is excreted through the kidneys. Negligible quantities are lost in the stool, sweat, and saliva. Lithium is filtered freely by the glomerulus. During each circulation of blood through the kidneys, one-fifth of the lithium ion filtered through the glomerular tubules is excreted in the urine; the remaining four-fifths is reabsorbed with sodium and water in the proximal tubules. Little or no lithium is reabsorbed in the distal tubules. Consequently, renal lithium clearance is about one-fifth of the glomerular filtration rate (GFR).

Individuals with normal renal function have a renal lithium clearance of 8 to 40 ml/min. (11, 12, 28). Renal elimination of lithium may be influenced by a variety of factors, including pregnancy, time of day, physical exercise, exposure to cold, sodium imbalance, and the administration of epinephrine (27). The mechanism underlying most of these changes is not known. In the absence of the above factors, there is usually little day-to-day or month-to-month variation in lithium clearance (22, 71).

Lithium clearance is independent of lithium's plasma concentration and is not significantly influenced by water loading.

There have been attempts to use measures of lithium excretion to identify potential lithium responders. Serry (29) conducted lithium excretion tests on a small series of manic patients and hypothesized that patients who excrete lithium more slowly than controls are responders, while those who excrete lithium more rapidly are nonresponders. Attempts to replicate Serry's findings have been unsuccessful (30), and it is now generally agreed that lithium excretion tests have little value as predictors of clinical response (14).

Metabolism

The lithium cation is not metabolized, although the accompanying anion may undergo metabolism. The anion, however, is pharmacologically irrelevant following absorption of the lithium salt and is important only as a vehicle for getting the cation into the blood and urine.

THE ELDERLY

Pharmacokinetics

With conventional lithium formulations, absorption and distribution are not significant sources of interindividual variance in pharmacokinetics or therapeutic effect. The major source of variance is the rate of excretion of lithium, more specifically, renal lithium clearance.

Since lithium is excreted almost exclusively through the kidneys, it would not be surprising if the drug's pharmacokinetics were affected by age. Age-related deterioration in normal renal function is well documented. In individuals with no renal disease, the glomerular filtration rate (GFR) decreases by about one-third between the third and eighth decades, with the greatest decline after age 60 years (24, 25). Renal plasma flow decreases by about 20%. Diodrast (radioopaque dye) clearance may be reduced by as much as 50%. The fall in GFR is of particular relevance for lithium therapy, since it can decrease the amount of lithium filtered through the glomerular membrane and reduce lithium clearance, thereby increasing the concentration of lithium in blood serum and tissues.

There is direct evidence that lithium excretion may be modified by age. Schou (26) reported that the average biologic half-life for lithium in patients over 60 years of age is approximately 36 hours, compared to an average half-life of 24 hours for middle-aged adults, and 18 hours for adolescents. At least part of the prolongation of half-life in the elderly is attributed to a decrease in glomerular filteration and lithium clearance.

Findings by Lehmann and Merten (18) tend to support Schou's contention that lithium clearance decreases with age. They compared a group of six middle-aged patients (mean age 58 years) to a group of ten young adults (mean age 25 years) and found a 60% lower renal lithium clearance in the older group. Fyro and coworkers (10), on the other hand, found no significant relationship between lithium clearance and age in a sample of 27 patients between 22 and 74 years of age. They contended that studies showing an age related decline in lithium clearance may have failed to exclude patients with renal disease, which could have adversely affected clearance. Clearly, there is need for longitudinal studies investigating the relationships among age, change in lithium clearance, and lithium tolerance.

Hewick (15), in an interesting study of 82 lithium-treated patients between 20 and 80 years of age, calculated the ratio of weight-related lithium dose to lithium steady-state plasma level for various age groups. The ratio remained constant over the third, fourth, and fifth decades and then declined over the sixth, seventh, and eighth decades. The ratio was about one-third lower in patients aged 70 to 79 years than in those aged 50 years. Part of this decline was attributed to an age-related deterioration in renal function. Hewick concluded that because of reduced lithium clearance in the older age groups, a lower lithium dose is required to achieve a given plasma level. However, Hewick cautioned that age alone can not explain the large variance among individual patients. Only 14% of the total variance in the ratio may be attributed to age. This suggests that individual differences in renal function within each age group are just as critical as differences generated by age per se. Fyro and coworkers (10), in their study of 27 patients of mixed age, also emphasized that there are large interindividual differences in the pharmacokinetics of lithium that appear unrelated to age. However, they did not offer any explanation for these differences.

Clinical and Therapeutic Effect

Although there are few systematic studies investigating the relationship between age and the clinical effects of lithium, there is general agreement in the literature that both therapeutic and toxic effects occur at lower plasma levels among the elderly. The elderly may be particularly vulnerable to confusion at lower blood levels. The confusion may be accompanied by neuromuscular irritability and imparied consciousness. This confusional state is a common sign of lithium toxicity in the aged. It can progress to coma and is often associated with continuing increase in blood lithium levels after lithium administration has been stopped. Even mild confusion may be troublesome, particularly where there is not close medical supervision. The patient's family may attribute the confusion to old age or senility, rather than to a drug-induced toxicity. As a result, the family may fail to seek medical help until the patient goes into a coma (27).

Another concern with lithium therapy in older patients is fine hand tremor. Lithium-induced tremor tends to occur more frequently in patients over age 60 than in patients under age 60 (26). Polyuria with increased thirst is also seen more frequently in patients over 60. There does not appear to be a critical plasma lithium threshold for either tremor or polyuria for any age group. Both reactions can occur at stable plasma levels of 0.6 to 1.2 mEq/liter (17).

The effects of lithium on thyroid function may also pose special problems for the elderly. Lithium inhibits the release of T3 (triiodothyroxine) and T4 (thyroxine) in the thyroid and may produce goiter or hypothyroidism. Serum T3 concentration may also diminish with age, exposing the patient to increased risk of lithium-induced thyroid pathology (32). In addition, hypothyroidism may simulate symptoms of dementia, which can delay appropriate treatment in the elderly patient.

Numerous dosing schedules designed to reduce the risk of toxicity in the elderly are reported in the literature. Some of the schedules use elaborate titration methods and test doses to determine vulnerability to toxic effects (29). Most seek a plasma lithium level of 0.4 to 0.6 or 0.7 mEq/liter (considerably lower than levels used with younger patients). These levels usually are achieved with doses of 600 mg to 900 mg per day. The usefulness of these schedules has not yet been adequately tested.

In sum, it is evident that patient age is a factor that must be considered in investigations of lithium pharmacokinetics and therapy and that lithium dosage may need to be markedly reduced in the elderly.

CHILDREN AND ADOLESCENTS

There is an increasing number of reports on the use of lithium with children and adolescents. These reports are difficult to interpret. There is no clear indication as to which childhood disorders respond to lithium therapy. Fragmentary evidence suggests that patients with periodic major disruption of mood and a positive family history of affective disorder are responsive to lithium (8, 33). It is also reported that lithium is effective in treating the symptom constellation of rapid mood changes, excitability, impulsivity, aggressiveness, and hyperactivity seen in a number of adolescents (5, 16). Unfortunately, the studies reporting these findings are characterized by small sample size, diagnostic heterogeneity, and lack of long-term followup. There is also an absence of studies comparing lithium against active medication or placebo.

In light of the above, it is difficult ot determine what constitutes an adequate therapeutic plasma level for children. There are reports that children and adolescents have a higher renal lithium clearance than their adult counterparts and hence tolerate higher doses. (19, 27). This finding requires further study under controlled conditions. There are also preliminary reports that lithium may have an adverse effect on calcium metabolism in the young person (19). If true, this would make lithium an especially undesirable treatment for children under age 12. Lithium's suppressant effect on the thyroid gland may also be troublesome with children. Clearly, more research is required on the biochemical, endocrinologic, and metabolic effects of lithium before the drug is used for long periods with children and adolescents.

REFERENCES AND BIBLIOGRAPHY

1. American Psychiatric Association Task Force on Lithium Therapy (1975): The current status of lithium therapy: Report of APT Task Force. Am J Psychiatry 132:997–1001.
2. Amdisen A (1975): Monitoring of lithium treatment through determination of lithium concentration. Dan Med Bull 22:277–291.
3. Amdisen A (1977): Serum level monitoring and clinical pharmacokinetics of lithium. Clin Pharmacokinet 2:73–92.
4. Ananth J, Pecknold JC (1978): Prediction of lithium response in affective disorders. J Clin Psychiatry 39:95–100.
5. Annell AL (1969): Lithium in the treatment of children and adolescents. Acta Psychiatr Scand (suppl) 207:19–34.
6. Bech P, Thomsen J, Prytz S, et al. (1979): The profile and severity of lithium-induced side effects in mentally healthy subjects. Neuropsychobiology 5:160–166.
7. Davis JM, Fann WE, El-Yousef MK, et al. (1972): Clinical problems in treating the aged with psychotropic drugs. In Eisendorfer C, Fann WE, eds: Psychopharmacology and Aging. New York, Plenum Press, pp 111–125.
8. Dyson WL, Barcai A (1970): Treatment of children of lithium responding patients. Curr Ther Res 12:286–290.
9. Foster J, Gershell W, Goldfard A (1977): Lithium treatment in the elderly. J Gerontol 32:299–302.
10. Fyro B, Petterson U, Sedvall G (1973): Pharmacokinetics of lithium in manic-depressive patients. Acta Psychiatr Scand 49:237–247.
11. Fyro B, Sedvall G (1975): The excretion of lithium. In Johnson FN, ed: Lithium Research and Therapy. London, Academic Press, pp 287–312.
12. Geisler A, Schou M, Thomsen K (1971): Renal lithium elimination in manic-depressive patients—initial excretion and clearance. Pharmakopsychiatr Neuropsychopharmakol 4:149–155.
13. Greenspan K (1975): Tissue distribution patterns of lithium in affective disorders. In Johnson FN ed: Lithium Research and Therapy. London, Academic Press, pp 281–286.
14. Groth U, Prelwitz W, Johnchen E (1974): Estimation of pharmacokinetic parameters of lithium from saliva and urine. Clin Pharmacol Ther 16:490–498.
15. Hewick DS (1978): Patient factors influencing lithium dosage. In Johnson, JN, Johnson, S eds: Lithium in Medical Practice. Baltimore, University Park Press, pp 355–363.
16. Horowitz HA (1981): Lithium and the borderline adolescent. Am J Psychiatry (in press).
17. Johnson BB, Dick EG, Naylor GJ, et al (1979): Lithium side effects in a routine lithium clinic. Br J Psychiatry 134:482–487.

18. Lehmann K, Merten K (1974): Die Elimination von lithium in abhangigkeit vom labensalter bei gesunden und niereninsuffizienten. Int J Clin Pharmacol Biopharm 10:282–298.

19. Lena B (1979): Lithium in child and adolescent psychiatry. Arch Gen Psychiatry (special issue) 36:854–855.

20. Lithium Carbonate Package Insert—Prescribing Information for Eskalith (Smith Kline and French Laboratories), Lithonate (Rowell Laboratories, Inc.), and Lithane (Roerig Division, Pfizer Laboratories), 1975.

21. Ljungberg S, Paalzow L (1969): Some pharmacological properties of lithium. Acta Psychiatr Scand (Suppl) 207:68–76.

22. Platman SR, Rohrlich J, Fieve RR (1968): Absorption and excretion of lithium in manic-depressive disease. Dis Nerv Syst 29:733–737.

23. Prien RF, Caffey EM (1976): The relationship between dosage and response to lithium prophylaxis. Am J Psychiatry 133:567–570.

24. Rowe J, Andres R, Tobin J, et al. (1976): The effect of age on creatinine clearance in men: A cross-sectional and longitudinal study. J Gerontol 31:155–163.

25. Salzman C, Shader R, Pearlman M (1970): Psychopharmacology and the elderly. In Shader R, DiMascio A eds: Psychotropic Drug Side Effects: Clinical and Theoretical Perspectives. Baltimore, Williams & Wilkins, pp 267–279.

26. Schou M (1969): Lithium: Elimination rate, dosage, control, poisoning, goiter, mode of action. Acta Psychiatr Scand (Suppl) 207:49–53.

27. Schou M (1976): Pharmacology and toxicology of lithium. In Elliott HW, George R, Okun R, eds: Annual Review of Pharmacology and Toxicology, Palo Alto, CA, Annual Reviews, pp 231–243.

28. Sedvall G, Petterson U, Fyro B (1970): Individual differences in serum levels of lithium in human subjects receiving fixed doses of lithium carbide. Relation to renal lithium clearance and body weight. Pharmacol Clin 2:231–235.

29. Serry M (1969): The lithium excretion test. Austal NZ J Psychiatry 3:390–392.

30. Stokes P, Kocsis J, Arcuni O (1976): Relationship of lithium chloride to treatment response in acute mania. Arch Gen Psychiatry 33:1080–1084.

31. Thomsen K, Schou M (1968): Renal lithium excretion in man. Am J Physiol 105:823–827.

32. Van Praag HM, ed (1978): Psychotropic Drugs. New York, Brunner Mazel.

33. Youngerman J, Canino IA (1978): Lithium carbonate use in children and adolescents. A survey of the literature. Arch Gen Psychiatry 35:216–224.

13

STIMULANTS IN THE ELDERLY

Carl Salzman

For nearly 30 years, central nervous system stimulants have been given to the elderly in an attempt to gain improvement in three types of function. These are

1. improvement of cognitive functioning, particularly short-term memory,
2. elevation of mood in the depressed older person, and
3. control of disordered behavior, usually agitation or withdrawal.

The results of research testing stimulants for these dysfunctions in the elderly have been disappointing for the following reasons:

1. Studies have usually focused on only one of these variables at a time. Studies negative for one, such as memory, may be positive for another, such as mood.
2. Measurement of cognitive performance is difficult and has not been standardized.
3. It is difficult to get patients to complete assessment instruments, particularly cognitive or behavioral.
4. Elderly patients may not take medications as prescribed; it is sometimes difficult to get very old people to take experimental medication at all.
5. Control samples are difficult to identify and recruit.

From the Psychopharmacology Research Laboratory, Harvard Medical School, Massachusetts Mental Health Center, Boston, Massachusetts.

Jarvik et al. (17) commented that there are no truly good, controlled studies of stimulant effects on cognitive performance in the elderly; furthermore CNS stimulants do not have a role in altering cognitive performance caused by organic pathology. Several studies have suggested that mild stimulants may alter declining social and interpersonal behavior. Stimulants may also play a minor role in improving depressed mood in the elderly.

Stimulants in the elderly have been the subject of at least five excellent reviews (2, 16, 19, 23, 24). Rather than comprehensively duplicate these reviews, this chapter focuses selectively on the role of CNS stimulants in treating impaired memory, mood, or behavior in the elderly. Five such drugs have received extensive study: (1) pentylene tetrazol; (2) pipradol; (3) pemoline; (4) amphetamine; and (5) methylphenidate. A sixth, piracetam, is a mild stimulant that tests have shown useful for memory (25). Because of its experimental status, it will not be included in this review.

These five stimulant drugs share the following characteristics (30):

1. All are psychomotor stimulants.
2. All increase stereotypic behavior and locomotor activity in the rat.
3. All are related to the phenylethylamine nucleus.
4. All stimulate the release of catecholamines and block their reuptake to varying degrees.
5. All are weak MAO inhibitors.

PENTYLENE TETRAZOL

Pentylene tetrazol has a long history of use as a circulatory and respiratory stimulant. It was used to induce seizures as a forerunner of electroconvulsive therapy and to counteract lethargy in patient recovery from illness and surgery. There are four theories regarding the therapeutic activity of pentylene tetrazol in the elderly:

1. facilitation of synaptic transmission,
2. stimulation of cortical psychomotor centers as well as brain stem vasomotor and respiratory centers,
3. enhancement of visual discrimination (in mice), and
4. reduction of circulating lactic acid.

There have been more than 50 studies of pentylene tetrazol in patients with chronic organic brain disease. The results have been mixed. Most positive studies only slightly favor pentylene tetrazol over placebo for improvement of behavior. Almost all report no effect on intellectual impairment, learning, memory, or motivation and attention for new learning (14). Jarvik et al. (17) believes the drug is most effective in facilitating learning in animals as the convulsive threshold is approached, making the drug dangerous for human use.

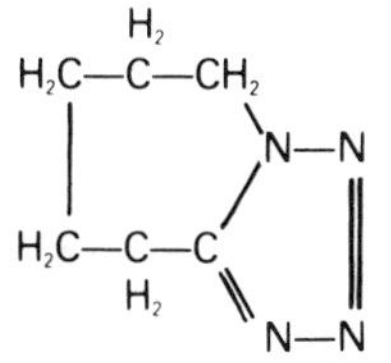

FIGURE 1. Pentylenetetrazol, a cortical stimulant sometimes combined with nicotinic acid. Sixteen controlled studies suggest it has a beneficial effect on geriatric cognitive function. Dose: 200 to 800 mg daily. Side effects: increased confusion, agitation, paranoid ideation.

There have been no studies of pentylene tetrazol on mood disorders, depression or pseudodementia, or apathetic behavior in the elderly.

Pentylene tetrazol is administered in a 200 to 800 mg dose daily, sometimes combined with nicotinic acid (see Figure 1).

PIPRADOL

Pipradol is a cyclized amphetamine derivative, with mild stimulant properties. It has been found slightly more efficacious than pentylene tetrazol for cognitive dysfunction, although it shares many of the same side effects (23). The theoretical bases for its effects are the following:

1. It increases central adrenergic activity.
2. It increases electrical activity in septal and hippocampal areas (18).

Pipradol does not significantly alter brain amine levels (32).

A 6-week study of pipradol in 68 patients, 50 years or older, found that 5 mg/day (as compared with 2 mg/day) decreased negativistic ward behavior without causing side effects (31). Alertonic, a geriatric elixir containing pipradol had no significant clinical or side effects (see Figure 2) (28).

FIGURE 2. Pipradol, a cyclized amphetamine and weak MAO inhibitor, with no appreciable effect on brain amines. It is in alertonic, which has no effect on geriatric mood or memory and no side effects.

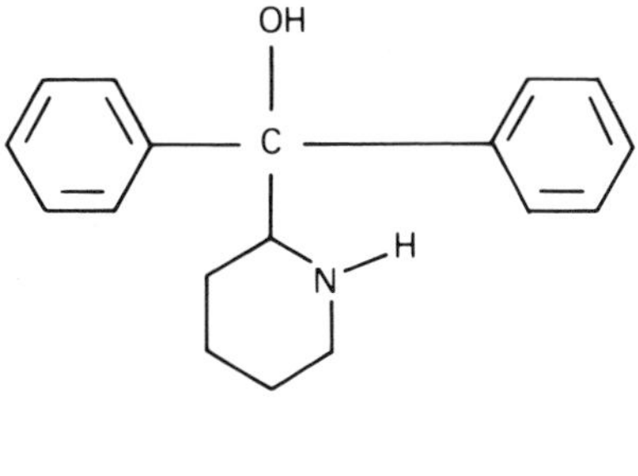

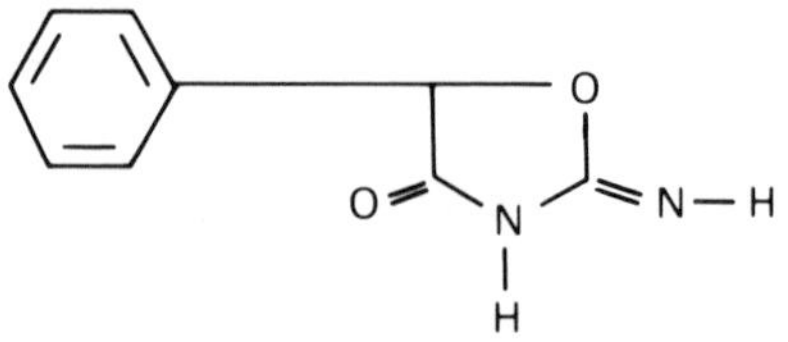

FIGURE 3. Pemoline, a cyclized amphetamine and weak MAO inhibitor. There are conflicting data on the effect on geriatric recall and learning.

PEMOLINE

Pemoline is a mild central nervous system stimulant with minimal sympathominetic properties (3). Although it had been hoped it would improve memory recall in older people (22) it has found clinical use primarily with hyperkinetic children (5). Pemoline was thought to improve memory by facilitating formation of RNA polymerase in rat brain (22).

In a 1-month, placebo-controlled study, elderly subjects given pemoline showed increased general interest and alertness. The authors concluded that pemoline was probably a CNS-arousing agent (9). A review of all pemoline studies in the elderly, however, concluded that pemoline had little overall clinical effect (32).

Results with pemoline are summarized in Figure 3.

AMPHETAMINE

For reasons of toxicity, amphetamines are little used clinically in the elderly. In addition to enhanced sensitivity to its CNS-stimulating properties, biologic alterations in the aging body alter the pharmacology of amphetamines. These changes associated with aging are the following:

1. Protein binding: Amphetamines bind to plasma albumin, although never in excess of 45% of the total drug (1). Plasma albumin concentration tends to decrease with age (27), which may predispose the aging person to higher circulating levels of free amphetamine.

2. Biotransformation: Amphetamines undergo para- and β-hydroxylation in the liver, the latter under the control of the enzyme dopamine β-hydroxylase (DBH). One study shows an increase in serum levels of DBH in people aged 41 to 60 years when compared with those 21 to 40 years old (12). However, a recent review of neuroendocrine aspects of aging does not report any studies of DBH levels in humans

past the age of 60, or in aged animal brain tissues (11). If DBH levels did decrease in aging humans, biotransformation of amphetamines would also decrease, with a resultant increase in toxicity.

3. Excretion: Sixty percent of amphetamine is excreted in urine within 24 hours and almost 90% within 3 to 4 days. Acidification of the urine decreases plasma elimination half-life. The ingestion of alkalinizing compounds, especially self-medication, a common practice in advanced age, may prolong plasma half-life and predispose to toxicity (29).

4. Drug interactions: Amphetamines interact with other catecholamine-increasing drugs or antihistamines, with resultant elevation in blood pressure. This increase may be well tolerated in the younger patient, but it may be disasterous in older patients with more fragile blood vessels, particularly in the brain.

5. Cardiovascular toxocity: Therapeutic doses of amphetamines may produce transient elevations in blood pressure (20). Furthermore, in the elderly person with diminished or impaired cardiac function, amphetamines may increase cardiac work excessively (14). For this reason, methylphenidate has been preferred as a CNS stimulant for older people. Despite potential toxicity, the therapeutic use of very low doses of amphetamines (5 mg BID) in younger patients suggest some potential usefulness in older people. Hackett (13) has reported amphetamines to be useful in certain clinical situations discussed below. Although he did not make specific reference to the elderly, these clinical conditions are also commonly encountered in advanced age.

   a. to decrease lassitude, in postsurgical and convalescing patients, especially in orthopedic patients with prolonged convalescence;

FIGURE 4. Amphetamine: Pharmacology. *Absorption:* Rapid and complete from all sites. Peak plasma concentration 1 to 3 hours after oral dose. *Distribution:* Binds to albumin in varying amounts. Never more than 45% of total drug. Drug concentrates more in tissues than in plasma. Large volume of distribution, mostly in kidney, liver, lung, spleen. *Half-life:* Twelve hours in man. *Biotransformation:* In liver via side-chain hydroxylation and deamination. *Excretion:* 60 to 65% in urine within 24 hours. About one-half is unchanged drug, one-half the deaminated metabolite. 90% excreted in 3 to 4 days.

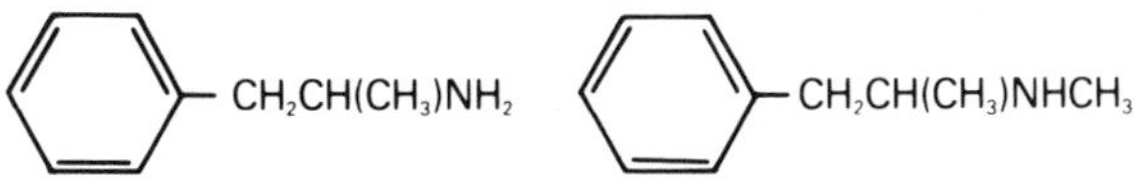

$CH_2CH(CH_3)NH_2$ $CH_2CH(CH_3)NHCH_3$

DEXTROAMPHETAMINE   METHAMPHETAMINE

b. to activate individuals who need to begin to socialize after a prolonged grief reaction following loss;
c. to improve mood and restore the sense of humor of terminally ill patients (1 to 2.5 mg);
d. to help in the differential diagnosis of pseudodementia. Cognitive impairment secondary to depression should improve with an amphetamine test dose.

The pharmacology of amphetamines is summarized in Figure 4.

METHYLPHENIDATE

Methylphenidate is a cyclized amphetamine derivative that decreases catecholamines from the reserpine-sensitive storage pool (21). It is absorbed orally with an elimination half-life of 3 hours. It is metabolized in the liver by biotransformation via deesterification. Methylphenidate inhibits cytochrome p450 reductase, which metabolizes tricyclic antidepressant (TCA) drugs. Therefore, when methylphenidate is given in combination with TCAs (a practice not generally recommended), increased TCA plasma levels result (33) (see Figure 5).

In one of the earliest positive clinical studies of methylphenidate in the aged, 62 negativistic apathetic patients over age 60 years were given a mean daily dose of 20 mg for 30 days (10). Positive improvement was noted in night behavior, socialization, cooperativeness, toilet and eating behavior, and decreased aggressiveness. There was no cardiotoxicity (10).

Subsequent studies reported conflicting results with methylphenidate and disordered behavior in the elderly. Recently, however, Kaplitz (18), in a placebo-controlled study, demonstrated beneficial effects of methylphenidate in 25 withdrawn, apathetic, geriatric patients. Drug recipients, compared with their placebo counterparts, showed improvement in ward behavior, interest, attention, involvement, and self-esteem. Competence, neatness, and psychomotor retardation all improved. These favorable

FIGURE 5. Methylphenidate: Pharmacology. *Absorption:* Complete via oral route. *Distribution:* Similar to amphetamine. *Half-life:* Three hours. *Biotransformation:* In liver via deesterification. Inhibits CP 450 reductase. *Excretion:* 50% after 8 hours, 90% after 48 hours.

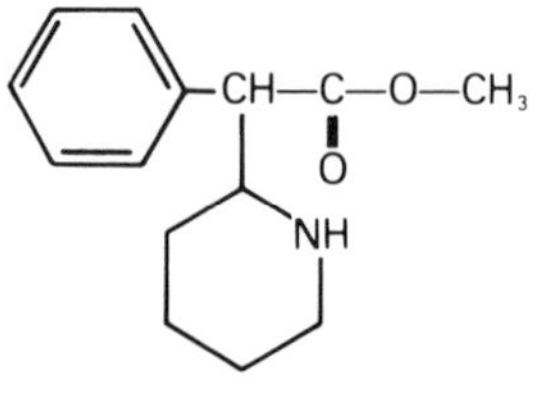

results led the authors to conclude that methylphenidate may be a useful substitute for pentylene tetrazol or tricyclic antidepressants.

The positive effect of methylphenidate on mood in the elderly was reported by Jacobson in 1958 (15) in a placebo controlled study. Twenty-seven patients, ages 60 to 70 years received 10 to 30 mg of methylphenidate for 2 to 6 months. Ten of the 27 patients showed moderate improvement in depression; no placebo recipients showed significant improvement. Davidoff et al. (8) also found methylphenidate useful in mildly depressed elderly patients, and Salzman and Shader observed methylphenidate to be a useful antidepressant for elderly females but not males (26).

Brannconnier and Cole (4) in a placebo-controlled study recently reported the results of a 42-day study of 60 fatigued, depressed, and mildly confused patients over 60 years of age. Twenty milligrams of methylphenidate was administered for 21 days and then increased to 30 mg for an additional 21 days with evaluations at 0, 21, and 42 days. Thirty-four of the patients who received methylphenidate experienced a decrease in depression as opposed to only 4% of those who received placebo. The authors concluded that methylphenidate improved depression, increased vigor, and decreased fatigue with only mild to moderate side effects.

Attempts to improve memory and cognitive function in the elderly with methylphenidate have proven less successful. In a placebo-controlled cross-over study, Crook et al. (6, 7) found that cognitive performance in the moderately impaired aged was not improved following administration of 10 or 30 mg of methylphenidate. At 45 mg, heart rate and blood pressure increased, but there was still no alteration in cognitive performance. In the study by Branconnier and Cole (4) confusion was not altered by methylphenidate and perhaps responded as well to placebo as to methylphenidate.

Overall, methylphenidate seems to have the following effects in the elderly (Table 1):

1. It shows less cardiotoxicity and less autonomic nervous system toxicity than amphetamines when doses are 30 mg or less daily.

TABLE 1. Methylphenidate: Activity

1. Cyclized derivative amphetamine
2. Increase tyrosine hydroxylase less than amphetamine
3. Releases dopamine from storage pool; blocked by reserpine
4. Mild MAO inhibitor
5. Beneficial for apathetic geriatric patients
6. No effect on cognitive functions
7. Dose: 20–30 mg daily
8. Side effects: increases in blood pressure and heart rate in aged subjects

2. It has little effect on cognitive dysfunction, when it is secondary to neuroanatomic changes in the CNS.
3. Methylphenidate is effective in decreasing depression, fatigue, and withdrawn behavior. Since cognitive functioning in the elderly may be impaired due to depression (i.e., pseudodementia or CNS under-arousal), cognition may respond secondarily to methylphenidate.

CONCLUSIONS

1. Stimulants are not useful for most cognitive problems of the elderly.
2. Stimulants have use in activating the withdrawn elderly person; they may also increase motivation for learning.
3. Stimulants are less effective in patients the more elderly they are, the longer their symptoms, and the longer they are institutionalized.
4. All stimulants have liability for cardiovascular and central nervous system toxicity, but methylphenidate appears to be the least toxic of the stimulants reviewed.
5. The clinical pharmacology of stimulants has been studied primarily in young adults. Extrapolation of these data to the elderly should be done with care. The metabolism of methylphenidate and other cyclized phenylethylamine stimulants in young adults is relatively rapid, as is excretion. Impairment of renal clearance, however, (an increased possibility in the elderly) may increase the risk of toxicity.
6. Unless the aging liver is severely damaged, metabolism (e.g., hydroxyla-tion and deamination) of stimulants should not be affected.
7. Decreased plasma proteins (primarily albumin) in the elderly have the potential for diminished binding of amphetamine.
8. Drug–drug interactions must be kept in mind when using stimulants. Stimulants in combination with other catecholamine-increasing drugs such as tricyclic antidepressants or monoamine oxidase inhibitors may increase the risk of serious cardiotoxicity, which could be disastrous in the elderly. Methylphenidate impairs the metabolism of tricyclic anti-depressants (TCA) leading to higher blood levels of the latter. In healthy younger adults, these elevated plasma TCA levels may be therapeutic; in the elderly they may be hazardous.
9. Methylphenidate is the most clinically promising of the stimulants. It should be studied in 30 mg/day doses for the following:
   a. differential gender response,
   b. age-related response,
   c. effect on "pseudodementia" or as a diagnostic instrument for pseudodementia, and
   d. use in chronic illness, convalescence, and grief or to restore humor.

REFERENCES AND BIBLIOGRAPHY

1. Baggot JD, Davis LE, Neff CA (1972): Extent of plasma protein binding of amphetamine in different species. Biochem Pharmacol 21:1813–1816.

2. Ban TA (1978): Vasodilators, stimulants and anabolic agents in the treatment of geropsychiatric patients. In Lipton MA, DiMascio A, Killam KF, eds: Psychopharmacology: A Generation of Progress. New York, Raven Press.

3. Biel JH, Bopp BA (1978): Amphetamines: Structure–activity relationships. In Iversen LL, Iversen SD, Snyder SH, eds: Handbook of Psychopharmacology, vol 1. New York, Plenum Press. pp 1–39.

4. Branconnier RJ, Cole JO (1979): The therapeutic role of methylphenidate in senile organic brain syndrome. Presented at Annual Meeting American Psychopathological Association.

5. Conners CK, Taylor E, Meo G, Kurtz MA, Fournier M (1972): Magnesium pemoline and dextroamphetamine: A controlled study in children with minimal brain dysfunction. Psychopharmacologia 26:321–336.

6. Crook TH, Ferris S, Sathananthan G (1977): The effect of methylphenidate on test performance in the cognitively impaired aged. Psychopharmacol bull 13:46–48.

7. Crook TH, Ferris S, Sathananthan G, Raskin A, Gershon S (1977): Effect of methylphenidate on test performance in cognitively impaired aged. Psychopharmacologia 52:251–255.

8. Davidoff E, Best JL, McPheeters HL (1957): The effect of Ritalin (methyl-phenidylacetate hydrochloride) on mildly depressed ambulatory patients. NY State J Med 57:1753–1757.

9. Eisdorfer C, Connor JF, Wilkie FL (1968): Effect of magnesium pemoline on cognition and behavior. J Am Geriatr Soc 23:283–288.

10. Ferguson JT, Funderbuck WH (1956): Improving senile behavior with reserpine and ritalin. JAMA 160:259–263.

11. Finch CE (1977): Neuroendocrine and autonomic aspects of aging. In Finch CE, Hayflick L, eds: Handbook of the Biology of Aging. New York, Van Nostrand, Reinhold.

12. Freedman LS, Ohuchi T, Goldstein M, Axelrod R, Fish I, Dancis J (1972): Changes in human serum dopamine-B-hydroxylase activity with age. Nature 236:310–311.

13. Hackett TT (1978): Use of stimulant drugs. Presented at the Annual Meeting, American Psychiatric Association, Atlanta.

14. Hollister LE (1975): Drugs for mental disorders of old age. JAMA 234:195–198.

15. Jacobson A (1958): The use of Ritalin in psychotherapy of depression of the aged. Psychiat Quart 32:475–483.

16. Jarvik M (1972): A survey of drug effects upon cognitive activities of the aged. In Eisdorfer C Fann WE, ed: Psychopharmacology and Aging. New York, Plenum Press.

17. Jarvik ME, Gritz ER, Schneider NG (1972): Drugs and memory disorders in human aging. Behav Biol 7:643–668.

18. Kaplitz SE (1975): Withdrawn, apathetic geriatric patients responsive to methylphenidate. J Am Geriatr Soc 23:271–276.

19. Lehmann HE, Ban TA (1975): Central nervous system stimulants and anabolic substances in geropsychiatric therapy. In Gershon S, Raskin A, eds: Aging, vol. 2. New York, Raven Press.

20. Martin WR, Sloan JW, Sapira JD, Jasinski DR (1971): Physiologic subjective and behavioral effects of amphetamine, methamphetamine, ephedrine, phenmetrazine and methylphenidate in man. Clin Pharmacol Ther 12:245–258.

21. Moore KE (1978): Amphetamines: Biochemical and behavioral actions in man. In Iversen LL, Iversen SD, Snyder SH, eds: Handbook of Psychopharmacology, vol 11. New York, Plenum Press, pp 41–98.

22. Plotnikoff N (1971): Pemoline: Review of performance. Tex Rep Biol Med 29:467–479.

23. Prien RF (1973): Chemotherapy in chronic organic brain syndrome—A review of the

literature. Psychopharmacol Bull 9:5–20.

24. Raskind M, Eisdorfer C (1976): Psychopharmacology of the aged. In Simpson LL, ed: Drug Treatment of Mental Disorders. New York, Raven Press.

25. Salzman C (1979): Update on geriatric psychopharmacology. Geriatrics 34:87–90.

26. Salzman C, Shader RI (1973): Responses to psychotropic drugs in the normal elderly. In Eisdorfer C, Fann WE, eds: Psychopharmacology and Aging. New York, Plenum Press.

27. Salzman C, Shader RI, van der Kolk BA (1976): Clinical psychopharmacology and the elderly patient. NY State J Med 76:71–77.

28. Shader RI, Harmatz JS, Kochansky GE, Cole JO (1975): Psychopharmacological investigations in healthy elderly volunteers: Effects of pipradol-vitamin (Alertonic) elixer and placebo in relation to research design. J Am Geriatr Soc 23:277–279.

29. Shock NW, Yiengst MJ (1950): Age changes in the acid-base equilibrium of the blood of males. J Gerontol 5:1–4.

30. Smith RC, Davis JM (1977): Comparative effects of d-amphetamine, 1-amphetamine, and methylphenidate on mood in man. Psychopharmacology 53:1–12.

31. Turek I, Kurland AA, Ota KY, Hanlon TE (1969): Effects of pipradol hydrochloride on geriatric patients. J Am Geriat Soc 17:408–413.

32. Weiss B, Laties V (1969): Behavioral pharmacology and toxicology. Ann Rev Pharmacology 9:297–326.

33. Wharton RN, Perel JM, Dayton PG, Malitz S (1971): A potential clinical use for methylphenidate with tricyclic antidepressants. Am J Psychiatry 127:1619–1625.

14

PHARMACOKINETICS OF NEUROLEPTIC DRUGS IN THE AGED

Thomas B. Cooper and Donald S. Robinson

Neuroleptic drugs are used in the aged to treat psychotic states associated with schizophrenia, schizoaffective illness, agitated depression, paranoid illness, and organic brain syndrome.

In general, the elderly are considered to be different from younger people in their response to drug therapy. While changes in drug metabolism represent a major potential source of age-related differences in drug response, the relative contributions of pharmacokinetics and pharmacodynamics to these differences have yet to be determined; this even though 21% of all first admissions to state and county mental health facilities in the U.S.A. are over 65 yr old (38).

The physiologic and pathologic changes that occur during aging may well accentuate the degree of variability found between individuals in their sensitivity to drug effects. The elderly who are mentally ill have a very high incidence (more than 80%) of concomitant physical illnesses (7, 58), which contributes to the high incidence of polypharmacy in these populations.

The use of drugs also increases significantly with age as does the incidence of side effects and drug interactions (27, 30, 37, 49). Ayd (6) in a study of a large number of patients reported extrapyramidal symptom disturbance in 50% of patients treated with neuroleptics in the age group 60 to 80 years. Psychotropic drugs may accentuate or initiate the clinical

From the Analytical Psychopharmacology Laboratory, Rockland Research Institute, Orangeburg, New York, and the Department of Pharmacology, Marshall University School of Medicine, Huntington, West Virginia.

Supported in part by General Research Support grant RR 05651-10.

picture of brain syndrome because of the elderly individuals' reduced cerebral reserve (38).

In a survey of drug induced deaths (excluding deliberate overdose) in Sweden between 1966 and 1970, psychotropic drugs were primarily involved in 9% of these deaths (total $n = 139$) (13). These data showed that the age-related incidence of untoward drug reactions remained reasonably constant up to age 50 years, after which a very sharp rise was seen (2 to 3 per 100,000 at 55 years, 15 to 16 per 100,000 at 70 years).

It is only in the last decade that chemical analytical procedures with sufficient precision and accuracy for assay of neuroleptic drugs in body fluids have become available. It is not surprising, therefore, that there is a relative paucity of data on the pharmacokinetics of these drugs in the aged. Several studies on the pharmacokinetics of other drugs in the elderly have recently been published (18, 28, 51, 57, 60), but with the exception of the review by Friedel (28) neuroleptic drugs are not discussed.

Shader and Greenblatt (57) emphasized recently that research in this area has progressed in two distinct directions, the first involving age-related changes in receptor sensitivity to drugs and the second involving age-related changes in pharmacokinetics. It is our task in this chapter to review the latter in terms of neuroleptic drugs only. We concur, however, with the statement of Shader and Greenblatt that "both of these research approaches are of importance at the basic and clinical levels and that an integrated research approach is most likely to provide meaningful answers to problems of drugs and aging" ([57], page 9).

AVAILABLE DATA ON NEUROLEPTICS IN THE AGED

Neuroleptic drugs are the most frequently prescribed drugs for institutionalized psychiatric patients. A comprehensive survey of the geriatric population of 12 veteran administration hospitals revealed that neuroleptic drugs were prescribed four times more frequently than any other psychopharmacological agent (50). Thioridazine was the most prescribed medication, accounting for 40% of neuroleptic prescriptions (50). Similar findings were reported previously by Altman et al. in a smaller study (2). This preference for thioridazine has been rationalized on the basis that for equivalent effective dosage, the incidence of extrapyramidal reactions is lower, and there is some evidence that dizziness and falling are less common (38). However, the incidence of nonspecific electrocardiographic changes associated with phenothiazine like compounds is disproportionally higher for thioridazine (16, 21). These effects are reversible and the pathologic significance, if any, is not clear at this time (38, 50). Despite this clear preference for thioridazine, controlled studies comparing thioridazine with other neuroleptics have not revealed any consistent differences in clinical efficacy or side effects in organic brain syndrome or schizophrenia (3, 61).

It is difficult to find descriptions of controlled studies specifically designed to compare the pharmacokinetics of neuroleptic drugs in the aged with a control population. Rather, groups of patients have been examined (usually in steady state with varying dose) with age included as one of the many variables of interest. The results of such studies have been (predictably) contradictory.

These data considered in the context of a rapidly increasing population of aged individuals (both proportional and absolute numbers) indicate clearly that there is a need for a thorough evaluation of the pharmacokinetics and pharmacodynamics of drug response in the elderly. The paucity of controlled experimental data on the pharmacokinetic aspects of neuroleptic drug response in the elderly makes a review confined strictly to the neuroleptics of questionable value. We have attempted therefore to relate what is known of the pharmacokinetics of the neuroleptics in general and of the other classes of drugs with similar physicochemical properties, to the few data on neuroleptics available from studies in the elderly in the hope that these observations may help stimulate well-designed research protocols in this area.

ABSORPTION

In the elderly there is a reduction in gastric pH, delayed gastric emptying, reduced intestinal blood flow and motility, and a possible reduction in the function and/or number of absorbing cells in the intestine (10). To date there is little, if any, evidence to suggest any major alteration in the absorption of neuroleptic drugs from the gastrointestinal tract. To our knowledge, however, there has yet to be a systematic study of a neuroleptic with the required rapid multiple blood sampling over the early period of absorption to address this question. The few pharmacokinetic studies on neuroleptics have focused more on the distribution and elimination profiles.

There is, however, a considerable amount of literature on the presystemic metabolism of the neuroleptics in the gastrointestinal (GI) tract and the effects on this metabolism of delayed gastric emptying. Thus, Curry et al. (19) demonstrated in an isolated guinea pig (ileum) loop experiment that only 15 to 30% of the chlorpromazine was absorbed unchanged. The intestinal microflora were much diluted in this preparation and it was therefore suggested that enzymatic degradation in the GI lumen in the intestinal wall was the logical explanation of this observation. In other experiments Hollister et al. (31) have shown that although the availability of oral chlorpromazine is markedly diminished (Figure 1)

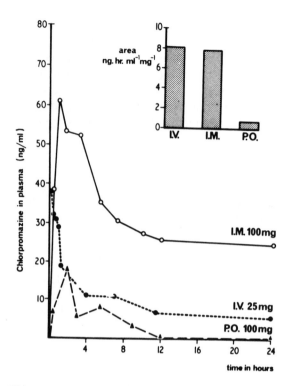

FIGURE 1. Chlorpromazine in plasma (nanograms per milliliter) and area under the plasma concentration time curve per milligram of dose following three doses in one patient. (Reproduced with permission from Sedvall, Uvnas, Zotterman, eds [1976]: Antipsychotic Drugs: Pharmacodynamics and Pharmacokinetics. Oxford, Pergamon Press.).

when compared to intravenous or intramuscular injection, the availability of the drug as determined by urine balance studies is very similar, indicating that the metabolites of the drug formed in the GI tract are readily absorbed. Rivera-Calimlim et al. (53) have recently demonstrated that lithium delays gastric emptying. Further, when normal volunteers were given single doses of chlorpromazine (100 mg orally), with and without lithium, lithium treatment resulted in a markedly decreased availability of chlorpromazine as determined by blood level curves of the parent compound. Similarly, Hollister et al. (31) compared various formulations of chlorpromazine and found that a spansule formulation resulted in essentially nondetectable plasma levels of chlorpromazine. This finding was again ascribed to extensive presystemic metabolism caused by the slow release characteristics of the formulation.

A number of factors combine in the elderly that may result in extensive drug metabolism both in the GI lumen, intestinal wall, and possibly by microflora of the GI tract (55) before the drug enters the portal system. These include delayed gastric emptying and decreased intestinal motility and blood flow. The use of drugs with potent anticholinergic activity (neuroleptic and antiparkinson) that inhibit gut activity and gastric emptying may compound these effects. The metabolites thus formed are readily absorbed (31) and may account in part for the increased frequency and severity of side effects in geriatric patients. An excellent source of data on alterations in gastric emptying caused by drugs and disease is a review by Nimmo (44).

DISTRIBUTION

Older patients tend to be smaller than younger people and therefore dosing without due regard to body weight may, in itself, lead to higher plasma and tissue levels. The elderly, however, often show elevated plasma drug concentrations that cannot be accounted for solely by changes in body weight (40). At the same time, significant changes in body composition do occur with age. Total body water decreases with age (22). Much of the metabolically active tissue is replaced by fat, body fat increasing from 18 to 36% of body weight in men and from 33 to 48% in women as they age from 18 to 55 years (45). Cardiac output decreases approximately 1% per year from age 19 to 86 years (11), and preferential distribution of blood to brain, heart, and muscle results in decreased hepatic and renal blood flow. Another aspect of distribution that requires clarification in the maintenance of the integrity of the blood–brain barrier to metabolites of these drugs. Drugs that act on both central and peripheral nervous systems generally show significant changes with age in their central effects, whereas their peripheral effects remain unchanged (12). Bender (9) has suggested that the increased toxicity of morphine in aging rats is the result of increased permeability of the blood–brain barrier. If this is so for neuroleptics in human beings, the possibility of psychoactive polar metabolites penetrating the blood–brain barrier and exerting profound central effects must be considered. However, there are few data available on age related changes in the blood brain barrier (see Chapter 2). The much-quoted clinical consensus that elderly patients are "more sensitive" to these medications (8, 23, 24) could possibly explain such a mechanism that would not necessarily be manifest by changes in the pharmacokinetic profile of the parent compound in plasma.

An additional aspect of drug distribution has been investigation of binding of drugs by red cells. Work by Chan et al. (15) demonstrated that red cell binding of pethidine in young patients was greater than that in the elderly and suggested such differences would explain the higher serum levels found in the latter group. Alfredsson et al. (1) have demonstrated rapid equilibration of chlorpromazine between plasma and erythrocytes of patients given chlorpromazine in single-dose studies. Manian et al. (41) have demonstrated that the phenothiazine drugs have a high affinity for the red cell membrane and that chlorpromazine and perphenazine demonstrate similar types of binding affinities in the red cell as in the rat brain synaptosomes. These observations prompted these investigators to suggest that red cell binding may be the mechanism by which the drug is transported to receptor sites in the central nervous system.

Finally, the recent demonstration of the importance of the alpha-1 acidic glycoprotein (orosmucoid) by Piafsky and Borga (47) in the binding of these basic lipophyllic drugs requires careful evaluation in the aged. These investigators have published a detailed study of chlorpromazine free drug levels in normal and various disease states and related these changes to the plasma alpha-1 acid glycoprotein level (48). It may well be that this acute phase reactive protein may vary considerably intraindividually because of the disease processes to which the aged are more susceptible, and this in turn may cause perturbations in the steady-state system, e.g., absolute increases and decreases in protein binding in the same patient.

ELIMINATION

Kato et al. (32, 33, 34) have demonstrated that hepatic microsomal enzyme activity is reduced in aged rats. Furthermore the liver mass/body weight, and cytochrome P_{450} content of the liver is reduced. Finally the induction response following treatment with phenobarbitone was also reduced. Swift et al. (59) demonstrated, in human subjects, a decrease in liver mass/body weight, an age related fall in antipyrine clearance, and some evidence for a reduction in drug metabolizing capacity per unit of functional hepatic parenchymal mass. An age-related fall in antipyrine clearance had been reported previously by O'Malley et al. (46).

The neuroleptic drugs are extensively metabolized in the liver, and the observations just noted in animals and human beings make it tempting to explain the higher drug plasma levels obtained in the elderly to diminished functional ability of the liver resulting in a prolonged elimination half-life and an increased pseudo-steady-state level. The cause of an increase in elimination half life, however, can depend on several interrelated variables other than the activity of hepatic drug metabolizing enzymes. The mathematical aspects of the pharmacokinetics of drug metabolism in the aged and interpretation of same have been recently presented by Gillette (29) and elsewhere in this volume by Wilkinson (see Chapter 1).

The few reports of the use of neuroleptics in older patients show increased steady state plasma levels even when normalized to a milligram per kilogram dosage schedule and occasional increases in the elimination half life have been reported. Few of these data have sufficient information to allow full pharmacokinetic analysis. Thus volumes of distribution are given in some studies but not in the context of aging. Plasma clearance or intrinsic clearance have not been measured in these studies, and thus whether the elimination half-life is increased because of reduced hepatic metabolism, volume of distribution changes or a combination of factors cannot be determined. A classic example of such possibilities is to be found in the work of Klotz et al. (36). In intravenous dosing the plasma half-life of diazepam was increased markedly in the elderly (90 hours compared to 20 hours in young controls), yet the plasma clearance in these same subjects was found to be similar. The volume of distribution was found to be correlated positively with age, and this difference alone explained the elimination half life increase.

The elimination of the neuroleptic drugs is further complicated by the observation that autoinduction of enzymes in the gastrointestinal lumen, intestinal wall, and the hepatic microsomal enzyme systems has been demonstrated unequivocally (19). Sakalis et al. (54) observed that chlorpromazine levels gradually declined after 3 weeks on a fixed dosage schedule. Loga et al. (39) confirmed this observation using antipyrine elimination as a marker for hepatic metabolism (antipyrine is primarily metabolized by the liver). Similar observations using other neuroleptics over prolonged time periods have been reported (17).

Dahl and Strandjord (20) in one of the very few detailed pharmacokinetic studies in this area, compared drug-free patients single-dose area under the curve to the same patients treated chronically (33 days) and found that with chronic treatment patients had smaller areas under the curve. Increased hepatic metabolism did not seem to be the cause in this instance, however, in that the elimination half-life was not changed. Rather, increased apparent volume of distribution caused by a decrease in availability owing to extensive presystemic metabolism in the gastrointestinal lumen and intestinal wall was postulated.

Rivera-Calimlim et al. (52) have claimed recently that patients chronically medicated have very low plasma levels of chlorpromazine when compared to drug-free acute admission patients. In an extensive analysis they postulated that plasma levels of chlorpromazine fall 10% per year on a fixed dosage schedule. We have observed such low levels in our own unit, and this can also be seen by examination of the literature in that chronic schizophrenic patients treated for many years with chlorpromazine and other neuroleptics rarely have elevated levels even when on very large doses, e.g., 1500 mg chlorpromazine/day.

Axelsson and Martensson (5) studied 169 patients with mixed diagnostic categories (103 females, 66 males) who had been receiving thioridazine for at least 8 days (age range 14 to 90 years). Of this total population, 141 were receiving additional medication. Forty-two patients were treated with thioridazine alone (age range 15 to 86 years) and had steady state plasma concentration measures. Twenty patients (age range 58 to 78 years) also had elimination half-life measures. There was no significant correlation between age and plasma concentration; however, the elimination half-life was positively and significantly correlated with age. It is of interest that in the entire group of patients ($n = 169$), plasma concentration was positively and significantly correlated with age. Yet these investigators were unable to demonstrate any significant difference between plasma levels of patients receiving thioridazine alone and those receiving additional medications. This is in contrast to the study of Buyze et al. (14), who demonstrated interference of additional medication on the plasma level of thioridazine, as did Muusze and Vanderheeren (43).

Martensson and Roos (42), in a study of 46 hospitalized patients (age range 17 to 89 years) who had been on a fixed dosage regimen of thioridazine (30 to 600 mg three times a day) for at least 2 weeks, found significant positive correlations in patients receiving less than 5 mg/kg between age and plasma concentration ($n = 22$). The reason for using 5 mg/kg as a cut-off point was that up to this level a strong correlation between dose and plasma level concentration was observed but above this dosage "the serum concentrations appeared to be randomly distributed." These investigators suggested that enzyme induction or anticholinergic effects may influence hepatic metabolism and gastrointestinal absorption. A similar observation with a cut-off of 6 mg/kg has been observed by Axelsson and Martensson (5). Klein et al. (35) have also reported a significant positive correlation between age and plasma level in a group of 18 schizophrenic patients. Muusze and Vanderheeren (43), however, in a study designed specifically to examine the plasma level and elimination half-life of thioridazine and metabolites in ten elderly psychiatric patients (age 56 to 78 years) were unable to demonstrate any relationship between plasma concentration and age. Axelsson and Martensson (4) studied the unconjugated thioridazine metabolite pattern in 212 psychiatric patients (mixed diagnoses), 130 of whom received other medications. A correlation was observed between age and metabolites in that elderly patients had significantly higher concentrations of thioridazine side-chain sulfoxide and sulphone. However, when other variables were included in the correlation as background variables these correlations were substantially weakened. Such findings warrant further detailed controlled studies in that changed metabolic profiles may indicate differences in enzyme activity, especially presystemic metabolism.

In extensive and detailed pharmacokinetic studies of haloperidol in 121 patients (mixed diagnoses), Forsman and Ohman (25) were unable to demonstrate any significant correlation between age and plasma halo-peridol correlation. These same investigators did find a positive correlation in a pilot study that involved patients of mixed diagnostic categories (26).

SUMMARY

The contribution of the various pharmacokinetic parameters of these drugs in the elderly will not be easily determined. The reduction in hepatic blood flow and liver mass may reduce intrinsic clearance which may be offset by extensive hepatic microsomal enzyme induction especially in chronically treated patients. The 45 kg 80-year-old woman who requires large doses of neuroleptic medication for adequate control of her symptomatology can be found in most psychogeriatric wards. However, the observations of reduced drug metabolizing capacity per unit mass raises the question whether hepatic microsomal enzyme induction could fulfill this role. Does increased presystemic metabolism then counteract this impaired hepatic clearance? If so, do these more polar compounds accumulate in the elderly because of reduced renal blood flow, is the blood brain barrier integrity compromised to the point that some of these normally excluded metab-olites penetrate the CNS or both? Does this mechanism explain sensitivity to drugs of the aged or is this age-related receptor site sensitivity? Are protein-binding changes resulting in changed kinetic parameters, such as volume of distribution, of clinical significance? Do disease states that increase the acute phase protein (alpha-1 acid glycoprotein), e.g., infection, inflammation, and cancer (56), cause clinically significant changes in the pharmacokinetics of these drugs?

Carefully designed controlled studies of these neuroleptic drugs addressing such problems specifically are most urgently needed. The past decade has seen the introduction of chemical analytical methodology with adequate precision and sensitivity to enable such experiments. When these data are available they will undoubtedly make a major contribution to the rational pharmacotherapy of the aged who are also mentally ill.

REFERENCES AND BIBLIOGRAPHY

1. Alfredsson G, Wode-Helgodt B, Sedvall G (1976): Original Investigations. A mass fragmentographic method for the determination of chlorpromazine and two of its active metabolites in human plasma and CSF. Psychopharmacology 48:123–131.
2. Altman H, Evenson RC, Sletten IW, Cho DW (1972): Patterns of psychotropic drug prescription in four midwestern state hospitals. Curr Ther Res 14:667–672.
3. Altman H, Mehta D, Evenson RC, Sletten IW (1973): Behavioral effects of drug therapy on psychogeriatric inpatients. I. Chlorpromazine and thioridazine. J Am Geriatr Soc 21: 241–248.
4. Axelsson R, Martensson E (1977): The concentration pattern of nonconjugated thiori-dazine metabolites in serum by thioridazine treatment and its relationship to physio-logical and clinical variables. Curr Ther Res 20:561–586.

5. Axelsson R, Martensson E (1976): Serum concentration and elimination from serum of thioridazine in psychiatric patients. Curr Ther Res 19:242–265.

6. Ayd FJ (1961): A survey of drug-induced extrapyramidal reactions. JAMA 175:1054–1060.

7. Bell WG (1973): Community care for the elderly: An alternative to institutionalization. Gerontologist 13:349–354.

8. Bender AD (1974): Pharmacodynamic principles of drug therapy in the aged. J Am Geriatr Soc 22:296–303.

9. Bender AD (1969): Geriatric pharmacology, Age and its influence on drug action in adults. Drug Ind Bull 3:153–158.

10. Bender AD (1968): Effect of age on intestinal absorption: Implications for drug absorption in the elderly. J Am Geriatr Soc 16:1331–1339.

11. Bender AD (1965): The effect of increasing age on the distribution of peripheral blood flow in man. J Am Geriatr Soc 13:192–198.

12. Bender AD (1964): Pharmacologic aspects of aging: a survey of the effect of increasing age on drug activity in adults. J Am Geriatr Soc 12:114–134.

13. Bottiger LE, Nordlander M, Strandberg I, Westerholm B (1974): Deaths from drugs. An analysis of drug-induced deaths reported to the Swedish Adverse Drug Reaction Committee during a five-year period (1966–1970), J Clin Pharmacol 14:401–407.

14. Buyze G, Egberts PF, Muusze RG, Poslavsky A (1973): Blood levels of thioridazine and some of its metabolites in psychiatric patients: A preliminary report. Psychiatr Neurol Neurochlr 76:229–239.

15. Chan K, Kendall MJ, Mitchard M, Wells WDE, Vickers MD (1975): The effect of aging on plasma pethidine concentration. Br J Clin Pharmacol 2:297–302.

16. Cole JO, Stotsky BA (1974): Improving psychiatric drug therapy. A matter of dosage and choice. Geriatrics 29:74–78.

17. Cooper TB (1978): Plasma level monitoring of antipsychotic drugs. Clin Pharmacokinet 3:14–38.

18. Crooks J, O'Malley K, Stevenson IH (1976): Pharmacokinetics in the elderly. Clin Pharmacokinet 1:280–296.

19. Curry SH, D'Mello A, Mould GP (1971): Destruction of chlorpromazine during absorption in the rat in vivo and in vitro. Br J Pharmacol 42:403–411.

20. Dahl SG, Strandjord RE (1977): Pharmacokinetics of chlorpromazine after single and chronic dosage. Clin Pharmacol Ther 21:437–448.

21. Dillenkoffer RL, George RB, Bishop MP, Gallant DM (1974): Electrocardiographic evaluation of thiothixene: A double blind comparison with thioridazine. In Forrest IS, Carr CJ, Usdin E, eds: The Phenothiazines and Structurally Related Drugs. New York, Raven Press.

22. Edelman IS, Liebman J (1959): Anatomy of body water and electrolytes. Am J Med 27:256–277.

23. Epstein LJ (1978): Anxiolytics, antidepressants, and neuroleptics in the treatment of geriatric patients. In: Lipton MA, DiMascio A, Killam KF, eds: Psychopharmacology: A Generation of Progress. New York, Raven Press.

24. Evans JG, Jarvis EH (1972): Nitrazepam and the elderly. Br Med J 4:487.

25. Forsman A, Ohman R (1976): Pharmacokinetic studies on haloperidol in man. Curr Ther Res 20:319–336.

26. Forsman A, Ohman R (1974): Some aspects of the distribution and metabolism of haloperidol in man. In Sedvall G, Uvnas B, Zotterman Y, eds: Antipsychotic Drugs: Pharmacodynamics and Pharmacokinetics. Wenner-Gren Center International Symposium Series 25. Oxford, Pergamon Press, pp 359–365.

27. Fracchia J, Sheppard C, Merlis S (1971): Combination medications in psychiatric treatment: patterns in a group of elderly hospital patients. J Am Geriatr Soc 19:301–307.

28. Friedel RO (1978): Pharmacokinetics in the geropsychiatric patient. In Lipton MA, DiMascio A, Killam KF, eds: Psychopharmacology: A Generation of Progress, New York, Raven Press.

29. Gillette JR (1979): Biotransformation of drugs during aging. Fed Proc 38:1900–1909.

30. Greenblatt DJ, Shader RI, Koch-Weser J (1975): Psychotropic drug use in the Boston area. Arch Gen Psychiatry 32:518–521.

31. Hollister LE, Curry SH, et al. (1970): Studies of delayed-action medication. V. Plasma levels and urinary excretion of four different dosage forms of chlorpromazine. Clin Pharmacol Ther 11:49.

32. Kato R, Chiesara E, Frontino G (1962): Influence of sex difference on the pharmacological action and metabolism of some drugs. Biochem Pharmacol 11:221–227.

33. Kato R, Takanaka A (1968): Effect of phenobarbitol on electron transport system, oxidation and reduction of drugs in liver microsomes of rats of different age. J Biochem 63:406–408.

34. Kato R, Vassanelli P, Frontino G, Chiesara E (1964): Variation in the activity of liver microsomal drug-metabolizing enzymes in rats in relation to the age. Biochem Pharmacol 13:1037–1051.

35. Klein HE, Chandra O, Matussek N (1975): Therapeutische Wirkung und Plasmaspiegel von Thioridazin (Mellaril (R)) bei Schizophrenen Patienten 8:121–131.

36. Klotz U, Avant GR, Hoyumpa A, Schenker S, Wilkinson GR (1975): The effects of age and liver disease on the disposition and elimination of diazepam in adult man. J Clin Invest 55:347–359.

37. Lamy PP, Vestal RE (1976): Drug prescribing for the elderly. Hosp Pract 11:111–118.

38. Lifshitz K, Kline NS (1970): Psychopharmacology in geriatrics. In Clark WG, del Guidice J, eds: Principles of Psychopharmacology. New York, Academic Press.

39. Loga S, Curry S, Lader M (1975): Interactions of orphenadrine and phenobarbitone with chlorpromazine: plasma concentrations and effects in man. Br J Clin Pharmacol 2: 197–208.

40. Luscombe, DK (1977): Factors influencing plasma drug concentrations. J Int Med Res 5: 82–97.

41. Manian AA, Piette LH, Holland D, Grover T, Leterrier F (1974): Red blood cell drug binding as a possible mechanism for tranquilization. In Forrest IS, Carr CJ, Usdin E, eds: The Phenothiazines and Structurally Related Drugs. New York, Raven Press.

42. Martensson E, Roos BE (1973): Serum levels of thioridazine in psychiatric patients and healthy volunteers. Eur J Clin Pharmacol 6:181–186.

43. Muusze RG, Vanderheeren FAJ (1977): Plasma levels and half lives of thioridazine and some of its metabolites. II. Low doses in older psychiatric patients. Eur J Clin Pharmacol 11:141–147.

44. Nimmo WS (1976): Drugs, diseases and altered gastric emptying. Clin Pharmacokinet 1: 189–203.

45. Novak LP (1972): Aging, total body potassium, fat-free mass, and cell mass in males and females between ages 18 and 85 years. J Gerontol 27:438–443.

46. O'Malley K, Crooks J, Duke E, Stevenson IH (1971): Effect of age and sex on human drug metabolism. Br Med J 3:607–609.

47. Piafsky KM, Borga O (1977): Plasma protein binding of basic drugs II. Importance of α_1-acid glycoprotein for interindividual variation. Clin Pharmacol Ther 22:545–549.

48. Piafsky KM, Borga O, Odar-Cederlof I, Johansson C, Sjoqvist F (1978): Increased plasma protein binding of propranolol and chlorpromazine mediated by disease-induced elevation of plasma α_1-acid glycoprotein. N Engl J Med 299:1435–1439.

49. Prien RF (1975): Genesis and treatment of psychologic disorders. In Gershon S, Raskin A, eds: The Elderly (Aging, vol 2). New York, Raven Press.

50. Prien RF, Haber PA, Caffey EM (1975): The use of psychoactive drugs in elderly patients

with psychiatric disorders: Survey conducted in twelve veterans administration hospitals. J Am Geriatr Soc 23:104–112.

51. Ritschel WA (1976): Pharmacokinetic approach to drug dosing in the aged. J Am Geriatr Soc 24:344–354.

52. Rivera-Calimlim L, Gift TE, Nasrallah HA, Wyatt RJ, Lasagna L (1979): Low plasma levels of chlorpromazine in patients chronically treated with neuroleptics. In Gottschalk LA, ed: Pharmacokinetics of Psychoactive Drugs: Further Studies, New York, Spectrum Publications.

53. Rivera-Calimlim L, Kerzner B, Karch FE (1978): Effect of lithium on plasma chlorpromazine levels. Clin Pharmacol Ther 23:451–455.

54. Sakalis G, Curry SH, Mould GP, Lader MH (1972): Physiologic and clinical effects of chlorpromazine and their relationship to plasma level. Clin Pharmacol Ther 13:931–946.

55. Scheline RR (1973): Metabolism of foreign compounds by gastrointestinal microorganisms. Pharmacol Rev 25:451–532.

56. Schmid K (1975): α_1 acid glycoprotein. In Putnam FW, ed: The Plasma Proteins. Vol. 1, New York, Academic Press, pp 183–228.

57. Shader RI, Greenblatt DJ (1979): Pharmacokinetics and clinical drug effects in the elderly. Psychopharmacol Bull 15:8–14.

58. Shanas E (1974): Health status of older people. Cross national implications. Am J Public Health 64:261–264.

59. Swift CG, Homeida M, et al (1977): A study of antipyrine kinetics in relation to liver size in the elderly. Br J Clin Pharmacol 4:730–731.

60. Triggs EJ, Nation RL (1975): Pharmacokinetics in the aged: A review. J Pharmacokinet Biopharm 3:387–418.

61. Tsuang M-M, Lu LM, Stotsky BA, Cole JO (1971): Haloperidol versus thioridazine for hospitalized psychogeriatric patients: Double-blind study. J Am Geriatr Soc 19:593–600.

III

OVERVIEW
AND FUTURE DIRECTIONS

15

GENERAL ISSUES RELATED TO AGE AND THE PHARMACOLOGY OF PSYCHOACTIVE DRUGS

Folke Sjöqvist

There are three main reasons to increase our knowledge of the influence of age on the pharmacology of drugs used in psychiatry: First, a deeper knowledge of the modifying effect of aging on the response to psychoactive drugs may broaden our understanding of brain function. Second, by defining specific alterations in pharmacokinetic processes in the elderly, better geriatric drugs may be designed. As an example, if a pathway of drug metabolism were to be impaired in the elderly, we would like to design drugs for geriatric use which are metabolized by other routes. Third, there is the ultimate hope that a better understanding of geriatric pharmacology may improve the use of drugs among physicians and patients. Although this is a highly desirable goal, it is very difficult to achieve. One example will suffice.

Inspired by the splendid research on drug use performed in the United States, we set out to develop systems for monitoring drug usage in Sweden in the late 1960s. One of these projects involves the county of Jämtland, where prescriptions to about 17,000 randomly selected individuals have been monitored since 1970 (9). In a representative part of the county it is possible to measure plasma levels of certain drugs in outpatients to assess their compliance with the prescription. The former project provides data on the drug, dosage, dosage interval, and sex and age of the patient so that

From the Department of Clinical Pharmacology at the Karolinska Institute, Huddinge Hospital, Huddinge, Sweden.

Many studies reviewed in this chapter were supported by the Swedish Medical Research Council (04X-3902, 29X-5015, 21X-5454).

the doses prescribed to different age groups can be compared. We were particularly interested in the prescription of drugs that are excreted unchanged in the urine for two reasons: (1) every doctor should know that creatinine clearance declines with age (14) and (2) most doctors should know that the renal clearance of creatinine usually parallels that of many drugs being excreted unchanged, such as digoxin (15, 22). One would therefore expect to find an age-dependent decrease in the doses prescribed of such drugs.

Using digoxin as a prototype drug we found that it was prescribed to 1585 patients in 1975 (8). The mean dose in the whole group was 0.21 mg daily. Compared to the middle aged, there was only a small decrease of the dose (from 0.23 to 0.20 mg) prescribed for patients older than 80 years (Table 1). Pharmacokinetic prediction based on age and creatinine clearance suggests that this age group should not receive higher average doses of digoxin than 0.14 mg (29), a rule of thumb supported by recent geriatric kinetic data (13). We found the same pattern of prescription for several other drugs being excreted unchanged. Thus, similar doses of tetracyclines, nitrofurantoin, and sulfonamides were used in the middle aged, in patients between ages 60 and 70 years, between 70 and 80 years, and in those older than 80 years. Continuing the investigation in the area where we could get blood samples, we found significantly lower plasma levels of digoxin than in age-matched hospitalized patients (5). Many old outpatients thus seemed to escape from the medical consequences of getting too high doses of digoxin prescribed by not taking it (29).

Reviewing the effects of aging on the kidney, Epstein (16) recently emphasized the need to take the 30 to 40% reduction in glomerular filtration rate in the elderly into account in drug prescription. Apparently we need better pedagogic methods to achieve this goal.

TABLE 1. Percentage Distribution of Prescribed Daily Doses of Digoxin in Different Age Groups in 1975 in the County of Jämtland, Sweden

| Daily dose (mg) | Age in years | | | | |
	15–59 $n = 125$	60–69 $n = 237$	70–79 $n = 773$	80+ $n = 454$	Total $n = 1585$
0.065–0.125	1	—	1	1	1
0.13	25	42	31	45	36
0.25	70	48	65	53	60
0.26–0.5	4	10	3	1	3
Mean	0.23	0.22	0.22	0.20	0.21

From Ref. (8).

DRUG EXCRETION

Psychoactive drugs (lithium excluded) generally have much more complicated kinetics since they are metabolized in the body before being excreted. I would nevertheless like to focus on drug excretion as my first clinical pharmacologic key word, for two principal reasons. First, the clearance of lithium is entirely dependent on kidney function, and one should therefore expect lower doses to be prescribed in the elderly. Second, some metabolites of psychoactive drugs are cleared by renal mechanisms. The possibility that these metabolites may accumulate in the elderly must therefore be borne in mind. Adverse drug reactions or enhanced clinical potency may result if the metabolites are pharmacologically active. As an example, impairment of cognitive function in uremic patients after amobarbital has been ascribed to the accumulation of the active hydroxymetabolite (4).

There is little quantitative information available on the renal clearance of hydroxylated metabolites of psychoactive drugs and even less on possible age dependency. Among the few examples to be found, unconjugated 10-OH nortriptyline has a renal clearance of about 80 ml/minute, compared to

FIGURE 1. Relationship between age and the ratio between 10-OH-nortriptyline and nortriptyline in plasma in patients treated with nortriptyline (solid circles) or amitriptyline (open circles). (Data computed from Ref. [7].)

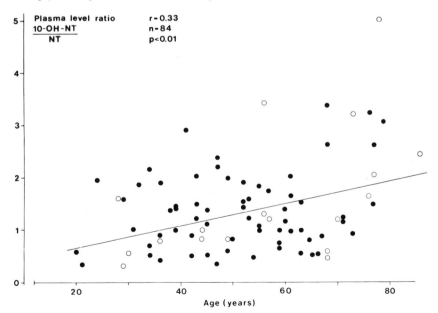

70 ml/minute for the conjugated form (24). One would therefore expect age dependency of the plasma concentration of this pharmacologically active (7) metabolite. Such a relationship, albeit weak, is indeed found as shown in Figure 1.

PHARMACOGENETICS

My second key word is pharmacogenetics, since the major source of interindividual variability in the kinetics of psychoactive compounds is differences in rates of metabolism (for a recent review see Ref. [28]).

Alexanderson (1) performed the first complete kinetic characterization of a psychotropic drug in twin volunteers using nortriptyline as a pharmacogenetic probe (23). He showed that the elimination rate constant (K_e), the apparent volume of distribution (Vd), and the plasma protein binding of nortriptyline were under separate genetic control. The interindividual variability in Vd and binding was small (less than twofold) compared to that in K_e (fivefold). Alexanderson (1) also showed that the plasma elimination rate constant of nortriptyline was related to the metabolism of the drug, assessed as the formation of the main metabolite 10-OH-NT.

The marked preexisting genetic variability in drug disposition (2) must be taken into account in the design of studies on the influence of age factors on kinetics. Often, the sample sizes used in such studies seem to be too small to ensure valid conclusions. The importance of using appropriate sample sizes is emphasized by the recent demonstration of a polymorphism in drug hydroxylation, the slow hydroxylator phenotype constituting only a few percent of the population (25). This is of interest in relation to the original demonstration of Hammer and Sjöqvist (21) that 2 of their 66 patients had steady-state plasma levels of tricyclic antidepressants far above those of the other patients. If a higher proportion of such outliers were to occur among the elderly, owing to selection factors, conventional statistical methods would be inappropriate to use in comparing elderly and controls. Moreover, a number of environmental, dietary, and disease factors likely to change with age may affect the kinetics of drugs (17, 32).

SELECTING DRUG SUBSTRATE

In studying the possible influence of age on drug metabolism, great care should be exercised in the selection of drug substrate. Ideally, the drug should have reproducible kinetics within an individual from time to time (implying minimal influences of environmental-dietary factors). Moreover, methods should be available to assess the unbound fraction of drug in plasma and to measure the major metabolite formed.

Braithwaite et al. (11) reported a slight age-correlated increase in steady-state plasma concentrations of nortriptyline (not significant) and amitriptyline (barely significant). Plotting literature data on nortriptyline kinetics they found the half-life increased with age while there was no significant decrease of plasma clearance. This brings up a fundamental pharmacokinetic point, i.e., that clearance (Cl_s) depends both on volume of distribution (Vd) and half-life ($t_{1/2}$). Thus

$$Cl_s = 0.693 Vd/t_{1/2}$$

An age-dependent increase in $t_{1/2}$ may therefore be caused by either decreased systemic clearance (the term reflecting rate of metabolism) or an increased Vd. Wilkinson (33) has discussed this problem elegantly using the benzodiazepines as examples (see also Chapter 1).

CLINICAL SIGNIFICANCE OF PHARMACOKINETIC FACTORS

There are also problems in interpreting the clinical significance of the reported age-correlated increases in steady-state plasma concentrations of psychoactive drugs (12, 20, 26, 31).

First, authors have not reported data on plasma protein binding. One may suspect that concomitant somatic diseases and changes in dietary habits may affect the concentration of plasma proteins in the elderly. As an example, alpha-1 acid glycoprotein, which binds basic amines such as

TABLE 2. Percentage Distribution of Prescribed Daily Doses of Nortriptyline and Amitriptyline in Different Age Groups in 1975 in the County of Jämtland, Sweden

Daily dose (mg)	Age in years			Total
	15–59	60–69	70+	
Nortriptyline	$n = 90$	$n = 25$	$n = 46$	$n = 161$
10–25	17	8	11	14
30–50	51	80	50	55
60–75	31	8	26	26
100–150	1	4	13	5
Mean	44	52	51	48
Amitriptyline	$n = 201$	$n = 129$	$n = 145$	$n = 475$
10–25	12	13	17	15
30–50	26	48	52	40
60–75	45	26	31	35
100–125	6	8	—	5
150–250	11	5	—	5
Mean	70	55	45	58

From Ref. (8).

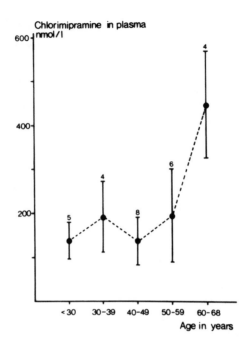

FIGURE 2. Relationship between age and total chlorimipramine in plasma. The levels correlated with age ($r = 0.51$, $p < 0.01$), but this is entirely due to the high concentrations in the four patients in the oldest age group. Mechanisms involved and clinical significance are obscure for reasons discussed in the text. (From Träskman et al. [31] by permission.)

antidepressants, phenothiazines, and β-adrenergic-receptor-blocking drugs, (27) rises in inflammation and malignancy. This will lead to decreased free fraction and increased total steady-state plasma concentrations per unit dose compared to patients with normal binding. However, neither clearance nor the unbound pharmacologically active drug concentration will change. Thus, there should be no enhancement of drug response.

Second, practically nothing is known about concentration-effect relationships for psychoactive drugs in the elderly (see below). Although there is a general notion that elderly patients are more "sensitive" to antidepressants, there are few hard data to support this contention. Studying the prescription of antidepressant drugs (the amitriptyline series) in different age groups we found some but no consistent reduction of dosage in the elderly (Table 2). The most striking feature was that the average doses prescribed to outpatients (50 mg) were very low regardless of age compared to those found to be effective in controlled clinical trials in hospitalized depressives (150 mg).

The overall impression given by the literature is that increases of steady-state plasma concentrations of certain psychotropic drugs with age occur but that they are difficult to evaluate in terms of mechanisms involved and clinical significance (Figure 2).

IMPORTANCE OF MEASURING DRUG RESPONSE

Finally, I wish to focus on the importance of measuring drug response in elderly patients. Many psychotropic drugs exert measurable effects on monoaminergic transmission in the peripheral and central nervous system. Investigations of monoamines and their metabolites in brain tissue in autopsy material show that changes occur with age (19). While the concentrations of dopamine and noradrenaline in different parts of the brain declined generally with normal aging, the changes of serotonin varied in different parts of the brain. Interestingly, Gottfries et al. (19) found that the levels of both homovanillic acid (HVA) and 5-hydroxy-indoleacetic acid (5HIAA) in brain seemed to increase with age. This apparent paradox was explained as the result of a reduced transport of these metabolites from cerebrospinal fluid.

It had been shown previously that the concentrations of both HVA and 5-HIAA in CSF increased with age (10, 18). In our own studies of depressed patients we have been able to confirm these findings using specific analytical techniques (Table 3).

These and other observations suggest that monoaminergic neurons may change their response to psychoactive drugs with age. The distinct possibility also exists that age-dependent alterations occur in the functional organization of drug receptors.

While age-dependent changes in the kinetics of drugs are relatively easy to measure there are considerable problems in recording the effect of psychotropic drugs in a reproducible way. This explains the paucity of data on the shape of concentration-effect curves for psychoactive drugs in

TABLE 3. Correlations between Amine Metabolic Levels in CSF, Age, and Height in Depressed Patients

	5-HIAA			HVA			HMPG		
	r^a	n^b	p^c	r^a	n^b	p^c	r^a	n^b	p^c
Age	0.32	84	0.003	0.51	39	0.001	0.44	44	0.003
Height (men)	−0.40	25	0.048	−0.52	14	0.058	−0.11	43	NS^d
Height (women)	−0.35	57	0.007	−0.55	24	0.005			

From Ref. (3).

[a] r, product moment correlation coefficient.

[b] n, number of patients.

[c] p, significance.

[d] NS, nonsignificant.

individual patients and in groups of patients including the elderly. Recent studies of the clinical pharmacology of antidepressants and phenothiazines show that it is possible to define their concentration-effect curves using biochemical endpoints such as changes in monoamine metabolites in cerebrospinal fluid (6, 30). These techniques are well suited for studies of the quantitative and temporal interrelationships between biochemical drug effects and clinical improvement and possibly also for elucidating age-dependent alterations in drug response under controlled kinetic conditions. It should be emphasized at this point that the relationship between concentration and effects of drugs such as antidepressants often deviates from the expected S curve. As an example, the relationship between steady-state plasma concentrations of chlorimipramine and the decrease of baseline CSF-levels of 5-HIAA is U shaped (31). Curvilinear relationships have also been found between plasma concentrations and clinical effects of other psychoactive drugs (28). The rating scales used to measure clinical improvement in psychiatric patients are probably not sensitive enough to assess the clinical consequences of any but the most pronounced age-dependent alterations in kinetics.

SUMMARY

The pharmacokinetics of drugs are known to change with age. The most unequivocal example is the decrease in renal drug clearance in the elderly. Yet few studies have been published on the elimination of potentially psychoactive drug metabolites in the elderly. Steady-state plasma concentrations of some psychoactive drugs seem to increase (per unit dose) with age, but the mechanisms involved are often difficult to evaluate since unbound drug concentrations have not been measured (33).

The clinical significance of age-dependent changes in pharmacokinetics cannot be assessed before the shape of the concentration-effect curve has been defined for each drug. A plea is therefore made for combining kinetic studies of psychotropic drugs in any age group with measurement of drug response using both biochemical and clinical endpoints. Such approaches are necessary to explore possible changes in drug–receptor interactions in the elderly.

REFERENCES AND BIBLIOGRAPHY

1. Alexanderson B (1973): Prediction of steady-state plasma levels of nortriptyline from single oral dose kinetics: a study in twins. Eur J Clin Pharmacol 6:44–53.

2. Alexanderson B, Sjöqvist F (1973): Pharmacokinetic and genetic studies of nortriptyline and desmethylimipramine in man. The predictability of therapeutic plasma levels from single-dose plasma concentration data. In: Pharmacology and the Future of Man, Vol 3. Basel, Karger, pp 150–162.

3. Asberg M, Bertilsson L, Thorén P, Träskman L (1977): CSF monoamine metabolites in

depressive illness. In: Depressive Disorders Symposia Medica Hoechst. Stuttgart, Schattauer Verlag, pp 293–305.

4. Balasubramaniam K, Mawer GE, Pohl JEF, Simons PJC (1972): Impairment of cognitive function associated with hydroxyamylobarbitone accumulation in patients with renal insufficiency. Brit J Pharmacol 45:360–367.

5. Bergman U, Sjöqvist F, Söderhielm L (1976): Use of digoxin in a low density population area in Sweden. Eur J Clin Pharmacol 10:19–24.

6. Bertilsson L, Åsberg, M, Mellström B, Tybring G, Sjöqvist F (1977): Factors determining drug effects in depressed patients—studies of nortriptyline and chlorimipramine. In: Depressive Disorders, Symposia Medica Hoechst. Stuttgart, Schattauer Verlag, pp 281–292.

7. Bertilsson L, Mellström B, Sjöqvist F (1979): Pronounced inhibition of noradrenaline uptake by 10-hydroxy-metabolites of nortriptyline. Life Sciences 25:1285–1292.

8. Boethius G, Sjöqvist F (1978): Doses and dosage intervals of drugs—Clinical practice and pharmacokinetic principles. Clin Pharmacol Ther 24:255–263.

9. Boethius G, Wiman F (1977): Recording of drug prescriptions in the county of Jämtland, Sweden. I. Methodological Aspects. Eur J Clin Pharmacol 12:31–35.

10. Bowers MB, Gerbode FA (1968): Relationship of monoamine metabolites in human cerebrospinal fluid to age. Nature 219:1256–1257.

11. Braithwaite R, Montgomery S, Dawling S (1979): Age, depression, and tricyclic antidepressant levels. In Crooks J, Stevenson I, eds: Drugs and the Elderly. Perspectives in Geriatric Clinical Pharmacology, London, MacMillan.

12. Collste P, Bergman U (1976): Significance of drug plasma levels based on the plasma level monitoring service of a department of clinical pharmacology. Arzeim Forsch 26:1255–1256.

13. Cusack B, Kelly J, O'Malley K, Noel J, Lavan J, Horgan J (1979): Digoxin in the elderly: Pharmacokinetic consequences of old age. Clin Pharmacol Ther 25:772–776.

14. Davies DF, Shock NW (1950): Age changes in glomerular filtration rate, effective renal plasma flow, and tubular excretory capacity in adult males. J Clin Invest 29:496–507.

15. Doherty JE, Flanigan WJ, Dalrymple GV (1972): Tritiated digoxin. XVII. Excretion and turnover times in normal donors before and after nephrectomy and in the paired recipient of the kidney after transplantation. Am J Cardiol 29:470–474.

16. Epstein M (1979): Effects of aging on the kidney. Fed Proc 38:168–172.

17. Gillette JR (1979): Biotransformation of drugs during aging. Fed Proc 38:1900–1909.

18. Gottfries CG, Gottfries I, Johansson B, Olsson R, Persson T, Roos BE, Sjöström R (1971): Acid monoamine metabolites in human cerebrospinal fluid and their relations to age and sex. Neuropharmacology 10:665–672.

19. Gottfries CG, Adolfsson R, Oreland L, Roos BE, Winblad B (1979): Monoamines and their metabolites and monoamine oxidase activity related to age and to some dementia disorders. In Crooks J, Stevenson I, eds: Drugs and the Elderly. Perspectives in Geriatric Clinical Pharmacology. London, Macmillan.

20. Gram LF, Reisby N, Ibsen I, Nagy A, Dencker SJ, Beck P, Petersen BO, Christiansen J (1976): Plasma levels and antidepressive effect of imipramine. Clin Pharmacol Ther 19: 318–324.

21. Hammer W, Sjöqvist F (1967): Plasma levels of monomethylated tricyclic antidepressants during treatment with imipramine-like compounds. Life Sci 6:1895–1903.

22. Iisalo E (1977): Clinical pharmacokinetics of digoxin. Clin Pharmacokinet 2:1–16

23. Kalow W, Inaba Y (1976): Genetic factors in hepatic drug oxidations, Prog Liver Dis 5:246–258.

24. Kragh-Sørensen P, Borgå O, Garle M, Bolvig Hansen L, Hansen CE, Hvidberg E, Larsen NE, Sjöqvist F (1977): Effect of simultaneous treatment with low doses of perphenazine

on plasma and urine concentrations of nortriptyline and 10-hydroxy-nortriptyline. Eur J Clin Pharmacol 11:479–483.

25. Mahgoub A, Idle JR, Pringle LG, Lancaster R, Smith RL (1977): Polymorphic hydroxylation of debrisoquine in man. Lancet 2:584–586.

26. Nies A, Robinson DS, Matthew J, Friedman J, Green R, Cooper TB, Ravaris CL, Ives JO (1977): Relationship between age and tricyclic antidepressant plasma levels. Am J Psychiat 134:790–793.

27. Piafsky K, Borgå O, Odar-Cedarlöf I, Johansson C, Sjöqvist F (1978): Increased plasma protein binding of propranolol and chlorpromazine mediated by disease-induced elevations of plasma α_1-acid glycoprotein. N Engl J Med 299:1435–1439.

28. Potter WZ, Bertilsson L, Sjöqvist F (1980): Clinical pharmacokinetics of psychotropic drugs—fundamental and practical aspects. In van Praag et al, eds: Handbook of Biological Psychiatry, New York, Marcel Dekker.

29. Sjöqvist F, Alván G, Bergman U, Boethius G (1979): Drug dosage in the elderly—theory and practice. In Crooks J, Stevenson I, eds: Drugs and the Elderly, Perspectives in Geriatric Clinical Pharmacology. London, Macmillan.

30. Sedvall G, Bjerkenstedt L, Nybäck H, Wode-Helgodt B (1978): The biochemical pharmacology of chlorpromazine treatment. In Tillement JP, ed: Advances in Pharmacology and Therapeutics, vol 7, Biochemical–Clinical Pharmacology. Oxford, Pergamon.

31. Träskman L, Åsberg M, Bertilsson L, Cronholm B, Mellström B, Neckers L, Sjöqvist F, Thorén P, Tybring G (1979): Plasma levels of chlorimipramine and its demethyl metabolite during treatment of depression. Clin Pharmacol Ther 26:600–610.

32. Vesell E (1979): Pharmacogenetics: Multiple interactions between genes and environment as determinants of drug response. Am J Med 66:183–187.

33. Wilkinson GR (1979): The effects of aging on the disposition of benzodiazepines in man. In Crooks J, Stevenson I, eds: Drugs and the Elderly. Perspectives in Geriatric Clinical Pharmacology. London, Macmillan.

APPENDIX
COMMONLY USED ABBREVIATIONS
AND ACRONYMS

AUC	=	area under the curve
BH_y	=	tetrahydrobiopterin or hydroxylase cofactor
BUI	=	brain uptake index
cGMP	=	guanosine-3; 5-monophosphate
Cls	=	clearance
CNS	=	central nervous system
CSF	=	cerebrospinal fluid
DBH	=	dopamine beta hydroxylase
5,7-DHT	=	5,7-dihdroxytryptamine
DMI	=	dismethylimipramine
DNA	=	deoxyribonucleic acid
DOPA	=	dihydroxyphenylalanine
GABA	=	gamma-aminobutyric acid
GFR	=	glomerular filtration rate
HDRS	=	Hamilton Depression Rating Scale
5HIAA	=	5-hydroxyindoleacetic acid
5-HTP	=	5-hydroxtryptophan
HUA	=	homovanillic acid
IMI	=	imipramine
kel	=	elimination rate constant
MAO	=	monoamine oxidase
MAOI	=	monoamine oxidase inhibitors
MBD	=	minimal brain dysfunction
MHPG	=	3-methoxy-4-hydroxyphenylglycol
NE	=	Norepinephrine

PCPA   = p-chlorophenylalanine
PKU   = phenylketonuria
PNMT   = phenylethanolamine-N-methyltransferase
RDC   = Research Diagnostic Criteria
$t_{1/2}$ = half-life
T3   = triiodothyronine
T4   = thyroxine
TCA   = tricyclic antidepressant
Vd   = volume of distribution

INDEX